**Milady's Standard
Cosmetology Exam Review**

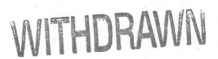

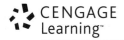

**Milady's Standard
Cosmetology Exam Review**

Edited by Elizabeth Tinsley

For product information and technology assistance, contact us at
Cengage Learning Customer & Sales Support, 1-800-354-9706

For permission to use material from this text or product,
submit all requests online at **cengage.com/permissions**
Further permissions questions can be emailed to

Library of Congress Control Number: 2002074216

ISBN-13: 978-1–56253–892–7

ISBN-10: 1–56253–892–6

Milady
5 Maxwell Drive
Clifton Park, NY 12065-2919
USA

Cengage Learning is a leading provider of customized learning solutions with office locations around the globe, including Singapore, the United Kingdom, Australia, Mexico, Brazil, and Japan. Locate your local office at: international.cengage.com/region

Cengage Learning products are represented in Canada by Nelson Education, Ltd.

For your lifelong learning solutions, visit
milady.cengage.com

Visit our corporate website at **www.cengage.com**

Notice to the Reader

Publisher does not warrant or guarantee any of the products described herein or perform any independent analysis in connection with any of the product information contained herein. Publisher does not assume, and expressly disclaims, any obligation to obtain and include information other than that provided to it by the manufacturer. The reader is expressly warned to consider and adopt all safety precautions that might be indicated by the activities described herein and to avoid all potential hazards. By following the instructions contained herein, the reader willingly assumes all risks in connection with such instructions. The publisher makes no representations or warranties of any kind, including but not limited to, the warranties of fitness for particular purpose or merchantability, nor are any such representations implied with respect to the material set forth herein, and the publisher takes no responsibility with respect to such material. The publisher shall not be liable for any special, consequential, or exemplary damages resulting, in whole or part, from the readers' use of, or reliance upon, this material.

Printed in Canada
14 15 16 17 12 11 10 09

Milady's Standard Cosmetology Exam Review

Edited by Elizabeth Tinsley

CENGAGE
Learning

Australia   Canad'   ‒ United States

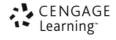

Foreword

Milady's Standard Cosmetology Exam Review has been rewritten to follow very closely the type of questions most frequently used by regulatory agencies, conducted under the auspices of the National-Interstate Council of State Boards of Cosmetology.

This review book is designed to be of major assistance to students in preparing for the various license examinations. In addition, its regular use in the classroom will serve as an important aid in the understanding of all subjects taught in cosmetology schools and required in the practice of cosmetology.

The exclusive concentration on multiple-choice test items reflects the fact that all theory licensure examinations are confined to this type of question.

Questions on the various examinations in different regions will not be exactly like these and may not touch upon all the information covered in this review. But students who diligently study and practice their work as taught in the classroom and who use this book for test preparation and review should receive higher grades on both classroom and license examinations.

Contents

History of Cosmetology

1. The Greek word kosmetikos means:
    a) skilled in the use of cosmetics
    b) trained in barbering
    c) skilled in hair care
    d) licensed to practice cosmetology

    _____

2. Haircutting and hairstyling have been practiced since:
    a) the glacial age
    b) the Golden Age of Greece
    c) the Renaissance
    d) medieval times

    _____

3. The first people to use cosmetics were the:
    a) Mayans
    b) Vikings
    c) Celts
    d) Egyptians

    _____

4. Henna is a dye extracted from:
    a) rose petals
    b) walnut shells
    c) dried bodies of insects
    d) the leaves of an ornamental shrub

    _____

5. Nail care was first practiced before 3000 B.C. in:
    a) Egypt and China
    b) Northern Europe
    c) India
    d) The Americas

    _____

6. Women in ancient Rome used hair color to indicate:
    a) how many children they had
    b) their class in society
    c) their marital status
    d) their religion

    _____

7. When monks and priests were forbidden by Pope Alexander III to shed blood, they enlisted the help of:
   a) barbers
   b) farmers
   c) servants
   d) carpenters _____

8. The barber pole, symbol of the barber-surgeon, has its roots in the early practice of:
   a) tooth-pulling
   b) bloodletting
   c) haircutting
   d) leeching _____

9. In 1875 the technique of using irons for waving and curling the hair was developed by:
   a) Charles Nessler
   b) Marcel Grateau
   c) Alexandre Godefroy
   d) Madam C. J. Walker _____

10. The first permanent wave technique that did not require the use of a machine was invented by:
    a) Evans and McDonough
    b) Charles Nessler
    c) Marcel Grateau
    d) Brisbois and Federmeyer _____

11. An important pioneer of the modern black hair-care and cosmetics industry was:
    a) Charles Nessler
    b) Sojourner Truth
    c) Marcel Grateau
    d) Madam C. J. Walker _____

12. An entry-level cosmetologist may be expected to perform a variety of duties, except for:
    a) selling retail products to clients
    b) updating client records
    c) paying bills
    d) making appointments _____

13. The first job a new cosmetology graduate is usually offered is:
    a) haircolor specialist
    b) salon stylist
    c) salon manager
    d) cosmetic chemist _____

14. A client desiring a new wave pattern will require the services of a:
    a) nail technician
    b) texture service specialist
    c) platform artist
    d) esthetician _____

15. Working with cancer patients who have suffered hair loss is a gratifying experience for a:
    a) haircolor specialist
    b) wig specialist
    c) nail technician
    d) texture service specialist _____

16. An esthetician can choose from many employment possibilities, including:
    a) massage therapist
    b) nail technician
    c) celebrity hairstylist
    d) consultant for a cosmetic company _____

17. To create a new image for a client, a makeup artist:
    a) performs a manicure
    b) uses cosmetics to blend and shade
    c) applies a body wrap
    d) provides haircolor services _____

18. A day spa offers the client:
    a) a full range of services
    b) massage therapy only
    c) esthetic services only
    d) health and nutritional services only _____

19. To be a successful salon manager, is it important to have:
    a) an eye for color
    b) styling skills
    c) creative talent
    d) the ability to supervise people _____

20. Product educators selling to professionals and salon owners often provide:
    a) product knowledge classes
    b) hairstyling techniques
    c) chemistry classes
    d) business training _____

21. A design team works together to present:
    a) new salon design
    b) regulatory issues
    c) new cosmetic products
    d) fashion and runway shows _____

22. The salon industry has grown tremendously and annually grosses :
    a) $50 million
    b) $50 billion
    c) $100 million
    d) $1 billion _____

23. Government regulatory agencies are involved in providing:
    a) continuing education
    c) trade publications
    b) standards for the industry
    d) job opportunities   _____

24. To develop your career to the maximum, it's important to:
    a) socialize with other
       cosmetologists
    c) always agree with your
       boss
    b) continue your education
    d) find your niche and stay   _____
       with it

25. There has been a huge growth in day spas, which offer many
    specialized treatments including all the following except:
    a) botox treatments
    c) aromatherapy
    b) nutritional counseling
    d) hydrotherapy   _____

Life Skills

1. A set of tools and guidelines for successful living is also known as:
   a) life skills
   b) prioritizing
   c) project management
   d) motivational drives
   _____

2. Building self-esteem is important because it:
   a) allows you to procrastinate
   b) ensures always being right
   c) makes you more important
   d) is vital to success
   _____

3. When you build a game plan you are:
   a) being compulsive
   b) consciously planning your life
   c) procrastinating
   d) wasting time
   _____

4. We can achieve greater control over our mental activity when we:
   a) procrastinate
   b) work long hours
   c) compartmentalize
   d) criticize ourselves
   _____

5. Motivation is an important factor in learning and usually comes from:
   a) interest in the subject matter
   b) a well-thought-out process
   c) a basic human need
   d) direction from others
   _____

6. When we feel self-love and acceptance, we have satisfied:
   a) emotional needs
   b) physical needs
   c) ethical needs
   d) social needs
   _____

7. Looking inward for new ways of thinking and doing is an example of:
   a) self-criticism
   b) creativity
   c) time management
   d) goal-setting
   _____

8. Writing a mission statement helps to establish:
   a) better communication
   b) understanding of others
   c) values and goals
   d) good technical skills
   _____

9. If a goal seems overwhelming, you can deal with it constructively by:
   a) dividing it into short-term goals
   b) changing your attitude
   c) lowering your goals
   d) procrastinating
   _____

10. When we practice time management, we can use a variety of methods, except for:
    a) taking time-outs
    b) making schedules
    c) prioritizing
    d) procrastination
    _____

11. One key to organizing time, a to-do list, can help you:
    a) prioritize tasks and activities
    b) become a systematic learner
    c) sharpen personal skills
    d) develop integrity
    _____

12. Identifying your learning style helps you to:
    a) respect others
    b) be punctual
    c) get along with others
    d) develop appropriate study habits
    _____

13. To stay focused on studying, it helps to:
    a) tackle the easiest task first
    b) keep your goals in mind
    c) allow distractions
    d) take no breaks until finished
    _____

14. The moral principles we live and work by are:
    a) honesty
    b) ethics
    c) goals
    d) character
    _____

15. A sense of integrity would prevent you from:
    a) talking too loud
    b) self-criticism
    c) stealing clients
    d) procrastinating
    _____

16. The code of ethics for the cosmetology profession is set by:
    a) state boards
    b) individual salons
    c) salon clients
    d) cosmetology schools
    _____

17. The following are all characteristics of good ethical standards except:
    a) cooperation
    b) honesty
    c) compassion
    d) punctuality
    _____

18. One trait that is essential to reaching the heights of professionalism is:
    a) ruthlessness
    b) commitment
    c) perfectionism
    d) good connections
    _____

19. Your attitude is a reflection of:
    a) good nutrition
    b) what you believe and think
    c) your communication skills
    d) your strengths
    _____

20. A healthy, good attitude includes many qualities except:
    a) good communication
    b) values and goals
    c) tactfulness
    d) perfectionism
    _____

21. Emotional stability allows us to:
    a) hold our feelings in
    b) express emotions appropriately
    c) manipulate all situations
    d) get our own way
    _____

22. If we understand the needs and motives of others, we are better able to:
    a) be prepared for anything
    b) take advantage of others
    c) act professionally
    d) stay isolated
    _____

23. An effective way to stay calm when under stress is to:
    a) hold in your feelings
    b) self-medicate
    c) take deep breaths
    d) avoid the situation
    _____

24. The best method when dealing with difficult clients is to agree with them and:
    a) call the manager
    b) ask another stylist to take over
    c) offer to remedy the situation
    d) tell them to file a complaint
    _____

25. As a cosmetologist you are perceived as a kind of caregiver, so it is important to:

a) take care of yourself

b) mix the personal and professional

c) ignore your own needs

d) give personal advice

_____

Your Professional Image

1. As a cosmetologist, your professional image consists of:
   a) technical skills
   b) good looks
   c) outward appearance and conduct
   d) sense of style
   _____

2. The Old English word hal means:
   a) hole
   b) house
   c) health
   d) whole
   _____

3. The key to a happy and productive life is:
   a) repressing bad feelings
   b) occasional exercise
   c) the latest diet
   d) achieving balance
   _____

4. Maintaining cleanliness and healthfulness every day is called:
   a) personal sense of style
   b) personal hygiene
   c) dressing for success
   d) personal grooming
   _____

5. One of the basics of personal hygiene is:
   a) daily exercise
   b) following the dress code
   c) daily bathing
   d) wearing perfume
   _____

6. The body's largest organ is the:
   a) stomach
   b) liver
   c) skin
   d) brain
   _____

7. In order to look well groomed at all times, the hair requires:
   a) regular shampooing
   b) blow-drying
   c) hair spray
   d) elaborate styling
   _____

8. The foundation of good personal grooming includes:
   a) a youthful look
   b) clean and cared-for clothing
   c) the latest styles
   d) a hip image
   _____

9. When choosing clothes to wear on the job, you must consider:
   a) your personal preferences
   b) the dress code of the salon
   c) the salon's color scheme
   d) the latest styles
   _____

10. When choosing your own hairstyle on the job, always take into consideration:
    a) your hair texture and wave pattern
    b) what your clients want
    c) your coworkers' styles
    d) the latest style
    _____

11. When applying makeup to go to work, it is best to:
    a) go for bright colors
    b) develop one approach
    c) apply it heavily
    d) accentuate your best features
    _____

12. As a beauty professional you are subject to many stresses, including all the following except:
    a) high expectations of clients
    b) standing on your feet all day
    c) the need to work faster
    d) 24-hour coverage
    _____

13. Establishing a routine for sleep, meals, and other daily requirements is:
    a) helpful in reducing stress
    b) a boring way to live
    c) unnecessary for the young
    d) difficult in today's world
    _____

14. In order to feel refreshed and eager to face the workday, it's important to:
    a) renew yourself with relaxation
    b) be punctual
    c) eat all you want
    d) seek medical advice
    _____

15. Good, nutritious food has many effects, including:
    a) preventing a variety of illnesses
    b) causing deficiencies
    c) putting on extra pounds
    d) causing chemical imbalances
    _____

16. Physical exercise has many positive effects on our bodies, including:
    a) lower immune function
    b) prevention of aging
    c) increased stress
    d) proper functioning of organs _____

17. Aerobic exercise, which improves heart function, includes all the following except:
    a) dancing
    b) yoga
    c) cross-country skiing
    d) walking _____

18. Physical presentation is an important aspect of professional image and includes all the following except:
    a) cleanliness
    b) posture
    c) an optimistic attitude
    d) good grooming _____

19. Among the guidelines for good posture while standing is to:
    a) keep the neck elongated
    b) let the shoulders drop
    c) tilt the hips toward the back
    d) keep the knees rigid _____

20. As a cosmetologist spending a great deal of time on your feet, proper foot care will help you:
    a) maintain good posture
    b) prevent carpal tunnel syndrome
    c) stay hydrated
    d) improve cardiovascular functioning _____

21. To increase blood circulation to the feet, try:
    a) tight socks or stockings
    b) foot massage
    c) jumping on a hard floor
    d) high heels _____

22. The science of "fitting the job to the person" is called:
    a) ergot
    b) ergonomics
    c) anatomy
    d) entomology _____

23. In order to avoid strain on your body when standing for long periods, consider:
    a) working with arms above shoulder level
    b) placing one foot on a stool
    c) wearing high heels
    d) slumping your shoulders _____

24. Among the recent ergonomic improvements to the salon workplace are:
    a) closely positioned workstations
    b) free-standing shampoo bowls
    c) low cabinets
    d) static chairs

    _____

25. To prevent physical strain, a good practice is to:
    a) hold arms away from your body
    b) swivel the client's chair
    c) twist your body when reaching
    d) grip implements tightly

    _____

Communicating for Success

1. Transmitting information through symbols, gestures, or behaviors is called:
   a) rituals
   b) communion
   c) communication
   d) sign language
   _____

2. When you communicate, you engage in all the following processes except:
   a) receiving messages
   b) meditation
   c) establishing relationships
   d) sending messages
   _____

3. An important first step in communicating with your client is:
   a) clarification
   b) advising
   c) making a sale
   d) giving your opinion
   _____

4. Repeating back to the client in your own words what you think she is telling you is called:
   a) repetition
   b) reflective listening
   c) mimicking
   d) impersonation
   _____

5. To determine the results your client is looking for, set aside time at the beginning of each appointment for a:
   a) gossip session
   b) gripe session
   c) client consultation
   d) personal discussion
   _____

6. During the client consultation, be prepared with certain items, including:
   a) pictures of yourself
   b) your diploma
   c) the salon's tardiness policy
   d) styling books
   _____

7. A person who prefers elegant, sophisticated clothing is categorized as having:
   a) a lack of imagination
   b) high expectations
   c) a classic style
   d) a large budget   _____

8. A client with young children who is not working outside the home will most likely choose:
   a) a layered style
   b) a dramatic look
   c) a low-maintenance style
   d) short hair   _____

9. Keeping thorough, accurate consultation cards for your clients helps:
   a) with reminder calls
   b) when you meet a new client
   c) build good client relationships
   d) keep your day on schedule   _____

10. When scheduling a new client:
    a) run a credit check
    b) allow extra time for a consultation
    c) call to be sure she's coming
    d) require payment beforehand   _____

11. Ideally, a special space should be set up for a consultation area and equipped with:
    a) salon supplies
    b) shampoo bowl
    c) hair color swatches
    d) old magazines   _____

12. If you learn during the consultation that your client does her own color services at home:
    a) refuse to work on her hair
    b) ask how often and with what products she colors
    c) offer to redo it for free
    d) laugh and shake your head   _____

13. One of the most important aids to use in your consultation is:
    a) food and drink
    b) a sales pitch
    c) shears and comb
    d) a mirror   _____

14. The best way to maintain the information gained during a consultation is by:
    a) recording it on a consultation card
    b) getting the receptionist to track it
    c) having the manager keep track
    d) asking the client to write it down   _____

15. The personal skills that will contribute to your success do not include:
    a) being honest and ethical
    b) smiling and being courteous
    c) giving others the benefit of the doubt
    d) always having the right answer   _____

16. If your client arrives past the limit for lateness, generally the best policy is to:
    a) let the client wait until you're free
    b) demand an explanation
    c) squeeze the client in
    d) ask them to reschedule   _____

17. The ultimate goal when dealing with an unhappy client is to:
    a) keep them from telling anyone else
    b) convince her that she's satisfied
    c) get her to pay for the service and return
    d) get her out of the salon   _____

18. One of the guidelines for dealing with a dissatisfied client is to:
    a) find out specifics
    b) tell her how great she looks
    c) suggest she give it time
    d) argue to prove you're right   _____

19. Calling on your manager for help with a client is:
    a) useful when all else has failed
    b) a bad career move
    c) the first thing to do
    d) potentially embarrassing   _____

20. In addition to developing good personal skills with your clients, it is important to:
    a) build relationships with coworkers
    b) avoid working with irritating coworkers
    c) keep all personal information to yourself
    d) share the latest gossip with your coworkers   _____

21. Guidelines for personal interaction with your coworkers include all the following except:
    a) sharing personal problems
    b) remaining neutral
    c) treating everyone with respect
    d) not taking things personally _____

22. Being objective with your coworkers:
    a) makes clients uncomfortable
    b) creates a cold atmosphere
    c) creates barriers
    d) cuts down on disagreement _____

23. One of the responsibilities of the salon manager is:
    a) getting involved in all issues
    b) looking out for stylists she likes
    c) keeping the business running smoothly
    d) resolving all personal problems _____

24. When having a problem with a coworker, approach your manager:
    a) as soon as the problem arises
    b) for help in solving the problem
    c) to get it off your chest
    d) to tattle on the coworker _____

25. To prepare for an employee evaluation:
    a) do a self-evaluation
    b) stay late
    c) flatter your manager
    d) cover up any mistakes _____

Infection Control: Principles and Practice

1. One-celled microorganisms with both plant and animal characteristics are known as:
   a) fungi
   b) cilia
   c) bacteria
   d) viruses
   _____

2. A type of pathogenic bacteria is the:
   a) saprophyte
   b) parasite
   c) virus
   d) cilia
   _____

3. Harmful bacteria are referred to as:
   a) nonpathogenic
   b) saprophytes
   c) protozoa
   d) pathogenic
   _____

4. Pathogenic bacteria produce:
   a) health
   b) beneficial effects
   c) disease
   d) antitoxins
   _____

5. A type of bacteria that lives on dead matter is:
   a) saprophytes
   b) flagella
   c) viruses
   d) parasites
   _____

6. Syphilis and Lyme disease are caused by:
   a) cocci
   b) spirilla
   c) diplococci
   d) bacilli
   _____

7. Cocci are bacteria with a:
   a) spiral shape
   b) round shape
   c) corkscrew shape
   d) rod shape
   _____

8. Bacilli are bacteria with a:
   a) corkscrew shape
   b) round shape
   c) spiral shape
   d) rod shape   _____

9. Bacteria that are arranged like a string of beads and cause strep throat and blood poisoning are:
   a) streptococci
   b) bacilli
   c) diplococci
   d) staphylococci   _____

10. Spirilla are bacteria with a:
    a) corkscrew shape
    b) round shape
    c) flat shape
    d) rod shape   _____

11. The bacteria that caused concern in 2000 in the pedicure industry was:
    a) Treponema pallida
    b) Pseudomonas aeruginosa
    c) Borrelia burgdorferi
    d) Mycobacterium fortuitum   _____
       furunculosis

12. The bacteria that rarely show active motility, or self-movement, are the:
    a) flagella
    b) cocci
    c) bacilli
    d) spirilla   _____

13. The slender, hair like extensions with which certain bacteria move about are called:
    a) spores
    b) flagella
    c) saprophytes
    d) diplococci   _____

14. Bacteria cells reproduce by simply dividing into two new cells in a process called:
    a) mitosis
    b) motility
    c) the vegetative stage
    d) the spore-forming stage   _____

15. During their inactive stage, certain bacteria, such as the anthrax and tetanus bacilli, form:
    a) flagella
    b) spores
    c) daughter cells
    d) toxins   _____

16. A communicable disease is:
    a) not transferred from one person to another
    b) prevented by vaccination
    c) transmitted from one person to another
    d) caused by nonpathogenic bacteria _____

17. A general infection, such as __, affects the whole body.
    a) a skin lesion
    b) syphilis
    c) a pimple
    d) an epidemic _____

18. Pus is a sign of:
    a) epidemic
    b) acquired immunity
    c) natural immunity
    d) infection _____

19. Viruses cause:
    a) tuberculosis and tetanus
    b) strep throat and blood poisoning
    c) abscesses and boils
    d) measles and hepatitis _____

20. One difference between viruses and bacteria is that bacteria:
    a) can live on their own
    b) become part of cells
    c) are resistant to antibiotics
    d) can penetrate cells _____

21. Hepatitis is a disease marked by inflammation of the:
    a) stomach
    b) kidneys
    c) heart
    d) liver _____

22. Acquired Immune Deficiency Syndrome (AIDS) breaks down the body's:
    a) digestive system
    b) skeletal system
    c) immune system
    d) nervous system _____

23. AIDS is caused by:
    a) the herpes virus
    b) poor personal hygiene
    c) the HIV virus
    d) contaminated food _____

24. The HIV virus can be transmitted by:
    a) sharing food
    b) kissing
    c) casual contact
    d) sharp implements _____

25. Bacteria and viruses can enter the body through:
    a) oily skin   c) broken skin
    b) dry skin   d) moist skin   _____

26. Molds, mildews, and yeasts are all:
    a) saprophytes   c) fungi
    b) viruses   d) bacteria   _____

27. In a cosmetology school or a salon, clients with contagious diseases and conditions should be:
    a) diagnosed and treated   c) referred to a physician
    b) sanitized and disinfected   d) given medications   _____

28. Resistance to infection is known as:
    a) immunity   c) immunization
    b) superiority   d) DNA   _____

29. Surfaces of tools or other objects that are not free from dirt, oils, and microbes are:
    a) contaminated   c) infected
    b) sterile   d) pathogenic   _____

30. Removing pathogens and other substances from tools or surfaces is called:
    a) scrubbing   c) autoclave sterilization
    b) decontamination   d) cleaning   _____

31. Sterilization is the only level of decontamination that kills:
    a) bacterial spores   c) the HIV virus
    b) both bacteria and viruses   d) tuberculosis bacteria   _____

32. Sterilization is used by:
    a) cosmetologists   c) surgeons
    b) housekeepers   d) nail technicians   _____

33. Surfaces that may be disinfected are:
    a) skin   c) nonporous surfaces
    b) nail plates   d) wood   _____

34. Disinfectants should never be used on human skin, hair, or nails because:
    a) they are not strong enough
    b) they may be drying
    c) damage can result
    d) they may stain skin _____

35. All disinfectants must be approved by each individual state and the:
    a) EPA
    b) OSHA
    c) MSDS
    d) FDA _____

36. Every product used in the cosmetology school or salon should have a/an:
    a) OSHA registration number
    b) warranty
    c) opaque container
    d) MSDS _____

37. Important information found on an MSDS includes:
    a) storage requirements
    b) resale value of product
    c) other suppliers of product
    d) other uses of product _____

38. OSHA was created to regulate and enforce:
    a) household accidents
    b) safety and health standards
    c) salon hazardous actions
    d) sanitary homes _____

39. A disinfectant that is "Formulated for Hospitals and Health Care Facilities" must be pseudomonacidal, bactericidal, fungicidal, and:
    a) easy to dilute
    b) inexpensive
    c) pneumonicidal
    d) virucidal _____

40. A salon implement that comes into contact with blood or body fluids should be cleaned and completely immersed in an EPA-registered tuberculocidal disinfectant or one that kills the:
    a) herpes and hepatitis virus
    b) HIV and AIDS virus
    c) HIV and herpes virus
    d) HBV and HIV virus _____

41. Any item that is used on a client must be disinfected or:
    a) given to the client
    b) discarded
    c) kept by the stylist
    d) washed _____

42. Before soaking in a disinfectant, implements must be thoroughly:
    a) soaked
    b) dry
    c) cleaned
    d) heated _____

43. Ultrasonic bath cleaners are an effective way to clean tiny crevices in implements only when used with:
    a) 70% isopropyl alcohol
    b) sodium hypochlorite
    c) an effective disinfectant
    d) an effective astringent _____

44. Most quaternary ammonium compounds disinfect implements in:
    a) 10-15 minutes
    b) 5-10 minutes
    c) 2-5 minutes
    d) 5-10 seconds _____

45. Phenolic disinfectants in 5 percent solution are used mostly for:
    a) skin sanitization
    b) rubber and plastic
    c) blood spills
    d) metal implements _____

46. Two disinfectants used in the salon in the past, but since replaced by more advanced and effective technologies, are:
    a) alcohol and bleach
    b) alcohol and quats
    c) phenols and bleach
    d) quats and phenols _____

47. States requiring hospital disinfection do not allow the use of __ for disinfection of implements.
    a) EPA-registered disinfectants
    b) quats
    c) alcohol
    d) phenols _____

48. The technical name for bleach is:
    a) sodium hydroxide
    b) sodium hypochlorite
    c) sodium chloride
    d) sodium hydroclorox _____

49. A product that is not considered safe for salon use because it causes a number of health problems is:
    a) alcohol
    b) bleach
    c) antiseptics
    d) formalin _____

50. Implements can be removed from disinfectants with any of these except:
   a) bare fingers
   b) tongs
   c) draining basket
   d) gloved hands
   _____

51. The solution used in a wet sanitizer should be changed:
   a) whenever it looks cloudy
   b) once a day
   c) every other day
   d) once a week
   _____

52. When mixing disinfectants, always:
   a) add disinfectant to water
   b) mix a weaker solution than recommended
   c) mix a stronger solution than recommended
   d) add water to disinfectant
   _____

53. Properly disinfected implements should be stored in a/an:
   a) disinfected and covered container
   b) open container at station
   c) station drawer
   d) wet sanitizer
   _____

54. Ultraviolet (UV) sanitizers are useful for:
   a) storing dirty implements
   b) sterilizing implements
   c) disinfecting implements
   d) storing disinfected implements
   _____

55. Linens and capes or drapes should be used once and then laundered with:
   a) bleach
   b) quats
   c) phenols
   d) antiseptics
   _____

56. Those parts of tools such as hair clippers that cannot be immersed in liquid:
   a) cannot be disinfected
   b) should be disinfected
   c) should be wiped with a wet towel
   d) should be rinsed quickly
   _____

57. Foot spas should be disinfected with an EPA-registered disinfectant with bactericidal, fungicidal, virucidal (and in some states tuberculocidal) efficacy:
   a) every two weeks
   b) once a week
   c) after each client
   d) once a day
   _____

58. Every two weeks, foot spas should be filled with __ that should be left to sit overnight.
a) a 5 percent bleach solution
b) an EPA-registered disinfectant
c) a 5 percent quat solution
d) hot soapy water _____

59. When disposing of contaminated wipes or cotton balls from a blood spill, they should be:
a) dropped into a trash can
b) double-bagged before disposing
c) wrapped in a towel
d) thrown into a Dumpster _____

60. The third, or lowest, level of decontamination is:
a) trash removal
b) disinfection
c) infection control
d) sanitation _____

61. Washing your hands is an example of:
a) sterilization
b) disinfection
c) sanitation
d) contamination _____

62. Rather than using bar soaps, which can grow bacteria, you should provide:
a) alcohol wipes
b) detergents
c) diluted bleach
d) pump-type liquid soap _____

63. In the salon, it is generally considered sufficient to wash the hands with:
a) plain water
b) EPA-registered cleansers
c) soap and warm water
d) disinfectants _____

64. The products known as antiseptics:
a) are classified as disinfectants
b) can safely be applied to skin
c) do not kill bacteria
d) are stronger than disinfectants _____

65. The guidelines and controls that require employer and employee to assume that all human blood and specified body fluids are infectious for HIV, HBV, and other bloodborne pathogens is called:
   a) HIV and HBV Guidelines
   b) Salon Precautions
   c) Disinfection Controls
   d) Universal Precautions   _____

Anatomy and Physiology

1. The study of the structures of the human body that can be seen with the naked eye is called:
   a) anatomy
   b) myology
   c) physiology
   d) histology
   _____

2. Living plant and animal cells are enclosed by the:
   a) cytoplasm
   b) nucleus
   c) protoplasm
   d) cell membrane
   _____

3. The substance of which all living cells are composed is called:
   a) protoplasm
   b) lymph
   c) leukocytes
   d) plasma
   _____

4. Food materials for cellular growth and self-repair are found in the:
   a) daughter cell
   b) cell membrane
   c) cytoplasm
   d) nucleus
   _____

5. The process of building up larger molecules from smaller ones is called:
   a) anabolism
   b) catabolism
   c) mitosis
   d) circulation
   _____

6. A tissue is a group of __ that perform a specific function.
   a) systems
   b) cells
   c) membranes
   d) organs
   _____

7. The brain and spinal cord are examples of:
   a) nerve tissue
   b) connective tissue
   c) epithelial tissue
   d) muscular tissue
   _____

8. The tissue that serves as a protective covering on body surfaces is called:
   a) nerve tissue
   b) epithelial tissue
   c) connective tissue
   d) muscular tissue

   _____

9. The heart, lungs, kidneys, stomach, and intestines are body:
   a) organs
   b) functions
   c) systems
   d) tissues

   _____

10. The circulatory system includes these organs:
    a) oil and sweat glands
    b) lungs and air passages
    c) stomach and salivary glands
    d) heart and blood vessels

    _____

11. The body system that serves as the physical foundation of the body is the:
    a) skeletal system
    b) nervous system
    c) respiratory system
    d) circulatory system

    _____

12. The scientific study of the anatomy, structure, and functions of bones is called:
    a) trichology
    b) biology
    c) osteology
    d) myology

    _____

13. The portion of the skull that protects the brain is the:
    a) cranium
    b) frontal bone
    c) mandible
    d) facial skeleton

    _____

14. An important function of bones is:
    a) producing red and white blood cells
    b) stimulating blood circulation
    c) stimulating the muscles
    d) producing calcium

    _____

15. The two bones that form the sides and crown (top) of the cranium are the:
    a) frontal bones
    b) temporal bones
    c) occipital bones
    d) parietal bones

    _____

16. The U-shaped bone that is commonly called the "Adam's apple" is the:
    a) nasal bone
    b) carpus
    c) mandible
    d) hyoid
    _____

17. The bony cage that serves as a protective framework for the heart, lungs, and other organs is the:
    a) scapula
    b) phalanges
    c) thorax
    d) sternum
    _____

18. The cheekbones are also called the:
    a) maxillae
    b) zygomatic bones
    c) lacrimal bones
    d) temporal bones
    _____

19. The largest and strongest bone of the face is the:
    a) zygomatic bone
    b) lacrimal bone
    c) maxilla
    d) mandible
    _____

20. The place where two or more bones connect is called a/an:
    a) tendon
    b) origin
    c) joint
    d) ligament
    _____

21. The temporal bones form the:
    a) lower jaw
    b) sides of the head
    c) forehead
    d) eye sockets
    _____

22. The bones of the forearm are the:
    a) phalanges
    b) ulna and radius
    c) carpus and metacarpus
    d) humerus and radius
    _____

23. The 14 bones in the fingers of each hand are the:
    a) phalanges
    b) clavicles
    c) carpals
    d) digits
    _____

24. The bridge of the nose is formed by the:
    a) frontal bones
    b) lacrimal bones
    c) nasal bones
    d) zygomatic bones
    _____

25. The place of attachment of a muscle to an immovable section of the skeleton is called the:
    a) belly
    b) origin
    c) insertion
    d) ligament
    _____

26. The study of the structure, functions, and diseases of the muscles is called:
    a) neurology
    b) osteology
    c) cardiology
    d) myology
    _____

27. The muscles that are attached to the bones and are controlled by the will are the:
    a) visceral muscles
    b) nonstriated muscles
    c) striated muscles
    d) cardiac muscles
    _____

28. The muscle that covers the top of the skull is the:
    a) procerus
    b) latissimus dorsi
    c) epicranius
    d) aponeurosis
    _____

29. The muscle that rings the eye socket is the:
    a) orbicularis oculi
    b) auricularis superior
    c) procerus
    d) orbicularis oris
    _____

30. The muscles of chewing or mastication are the:
    a) pectoralis major and minor
    b) zygomaticus major and minor
    c) buccinator and mentalis muscles
    d) masseter and temporalis muscles
    _____

31. One of the muscles that control the swinging movements of the arm is the:
    a) deltoid
    b) trapezius
    c) serratus anterior
    d) extensor
    _____

32. The muscle of the neck that lowers and rotates the head is the:
    a) pectoralis
    b) sternocleidomastoideus
    c) orbicularis oris
    d) platysma
    _____

33. The muscles that draw the fingers together are the:
    a) extensors
    b) opponents
    c) adductors
    d) abductors
    _____

34. The brain, spinal cord, spinal nerves, and cranial nerves make up the:
    a) autonomic nervous system
    b) circulatory system
    c) central nervous system
    d) peripheral nervous system _____

35. The largest and most complex nerve tissue in the body is the:
    a) fifth cranial nerve
    b) spinal cord
    c) spinal nerves
    d) brain _____

36. The sensations of touch, cold, heat, sight, and hearing are carried to the brain by:
    a) reflexes
    b) motor nerves
    c) sensory nerves
    d) efferent nerves _____

37. The part of the nerve cell, or neuron, that sends impulses away from the cell body to other neurons, glands, or muscles is the:
    a) spinal cord
    b) axon
    c) cell body
    d) dendrites _____

38. A branch of the fifth cranial nerve affecting the external ear and skin above the temple is the:
    a) auriculotemporal nerve
    b) infraorbital nerve
    c) mental nerve
    d) infratrochlear nerve _____

39. The point and lower side of the nose are affected by the:
    a) nasal nerve
    b) supraorbital nerve
    c) intratrochlear nerve
    d) supratrochlear nerve _____

40. The largest cranial nerve is the:
    a) mental nerve
    b) supraorbital nerve
    c) maxillary nerve
    d) fifth cranial nerve _____

41. The skin of the forehead and eyebrows is affected by the:
    a) infraorbital nerve
    b) supraorbital nerve
    c) infratrochlear nerve
    d) supratrochlear nerve _____

42. The chief motor nerve of the face is the:
    a) seventh cranial nerve
    b) supraorbital nerve
    c) fifth cranial nerve
    d) mental nerve _____

43. The nerve that affects the muscles of the upper part of the cheek is the:
    a) posterior auricular nerve
    c) buccal nerve
    b) temporal nerve
    d) zygomatic nerve
    _____

44. The muscles of the mouth are affected by the:
    a) mandibular nerve
    c) posterior auricular nerve
    b) buccal nerve
    d) zygomatic nerve
    _____

45. The nerves that originate at the spinal cord are the:
    a) radial nerves
    c) zygomatic nerve
    b) mandibular nerves
    d) cervical nerves
    _____

46. The cervical nerve that affects the front and sides of the neck as far down as the breastbone is the:
    a) lesser auricular nerve
    c) lesser occipital nerve
    b) greater occipital nerve
    d) cervical cutaneous nerve
    _____

47. The sensory motor nerve that, with its branches, supplies the thumb side of the arm and back of the hand is the:
    a) radial nerve
    c) digital nerve
    b) ulnar nerve
    d) median nerve
    _____

48. One of four principal nerves of the arm and hand that supplies the fingers is the:
    a) digital nerve
    c) ulnar nerve
    b) median nerve
    d) radial nerve
    _____

49. The steady circulation of blood through the body is controlled by the:
    a) circulatory system
    c) lymphatic system
    b) skeletal system
    d) nervous system
    _____

50. The blood-vascular system comprises the heart, arteries, veins, and:
    a) ventricles
    c) lymphatics
    b) capillaries
    d) atria
    _____

51. The upper heart chambers are called the:
    a) valves
    c) atria
    b) capillaries
    d) lymph
    _____

52. The interior of the heart contains the atria and the:
    a) valves   c) lymph
    b) ventricles   d) capillaries   _____

53. Vessels that carry blood away from the heart are called:
    a) capillaries   c) valves
    b) arteries   d) veins   _____

54. Vessels that carry blood to the heart are called:
    a) arteries   c) valves
    b) capillaries   d) veins   _____

55. The clear yellowish fluid that circulates in the lymphatics of
    the body is the:
    a) veins   c) plasma
    b) neuron   d) lymph   _____

56. The membrane that encloses the heart is the:
    a) atria   c) lymph
    b) pericardium   d) aorta   _____

57. Blood is composed of red and white corpuscles, platelets,
    plasma and:
    a) leukocytes   c) hemoglobin
    b) erythrocytes   d) thrombocytes   _____

58. The human body has eight to ten pints of the nutritive fluid
    called:
    a) platelets   c) leukocytes
    b) blood   d) plasma   _____

59. The fluid part of blood in which platelets and blood cells flow
    is:
    a) pericardium   c) thrombocytes
    b) plasma   d) hemoglobin   _____

60. Cells that contribute to the blood-clotting process are:
    a) plasma   c) white corpuscles
    b) platelets   d) red corpuscles   _____

61. Hemoglobin, which gives blood its bright red color, is found in the:
a) platelets
b) red blood cells
c) leukocytes
d) white corpuscles _____

62. One of the critical functions blood performs is:
a) keeping itself from clotting
b) varying the body's temperature
c) carrying nutritive substances to all body cells
d) carrying carbon dioxide to all body cells _____

63. Lymph is circulated through the lymphatic vessels and filtered by the:
a) leukocytes
b) platelets
c) lymph nodes
d) arteries _____

64. The brain, eyes, eyelids and nose are supplied blood by the:
a) external maxillary artery
b) internal carotid artery
c) parietal artery
d) external carotid artery _____

65. The artery that supplies blood to the upper lip and nose region is the:
a) inferior labial artery
b) superior labial artery
c) submental artery
d) angular artery _____

66. The external maxillary artery is also known as the:
a) superficial temporal artery
b) facial artery
c) occipital artery
d) posterior auricular artery _____

67. The artery that supplies blood to the temples is the:
a) anterior auricular artery
b) frontal artery
c) middle temporal artery
d) parietal artery _____

68. Two branches of the internal carotid artery that are important to know are the:
a) occipital and posterior auricular
b) supraorbital and infraorbital
c) anterior and posterior auricular
d) supraorbital and superorbital _____

69. The two arteries that are the main supply of blood to the arms and hands are called the:
    a) erythrocytes and leukocytes
    b) facial and external maxillary arteries
    c) internal and external carotid arteries
    d) ulnar and radial

    _____

70. The group of specialized glands affecting development and sexual activities is the:
    a) excretory system
    b) endocrine system
    c) digestive system
    d) circulatory system

    _____

71. The sweat and oil glands of the skin are:
    a) duct glands
    b) hormonal glands
    c) ductless glands
    d) endocrine glands

    _____

72. Insulin, adrenaline, and estrogen are all examples of:
    a) hormones
    b) digestive enzymes
    c) duct glands
    d) platelets

    _____

73. The digestive system is also called the:
    a) excretory system
    b) integumentary system
    c) gastrointestinal system
    d) respiratory system

    _____

74. The body system that enables breathing is the:
    a) endocrine system
    b) circulatory system
    c) excretory system
    d) respiratory system

    _____

75. The skin plays an important role in the excretory system because it eliminates:
    a) oxygen
    b) bile
    c) perspiration
    d) carbon dioxide

    _____

Basics of Chemistry and Electricity

1. Organic chemistry is the study of substances containing:
   a) carbon   c) hydrogen
   b) water   d) organisms   _____

2. Examples of organic substances include:
   a) pesticides   c) pure water
   b) minerals   d) metals   _____

3. Matter is any substance that:
   a) occupies space   c) is soluble in water
   b) contains carbon   d) is either a solid or liquid   _____

4. The particles from which all matter is composed are:
   a) elemental molecules   c) atoms
   b) compound molecules   d) chemical compounds   _____

5. Two or more atoms of the same element that are united chemically form a/an:
   a) elemental molecule   c) compound molecule
   b) chemical compound   d) state of matter   _____

6. When water boils, it is changing from one state of matter to another, from:
   a) liquid to gas   c) solid to liquid
   b) gas to liquid   d) solid to gas   _____

7. When a physical change occurs in a substance, there is:
   a) a change in physical   c) the formation of a new
      properties   substance
   b) no change in state of   d) a chemical reaction   _____
      matter

8. The action of permanent haircolor is an example of a:
   a) physical change   c) chemical change
   b) temporary change   d) change in state of matter _____

9. Water (H_2O) is an example of a/an:
   a) chemical compound   c) physical mixture
   b) element   d) solution _____

10. Salt water and fruit salad are examples of a/an:
    a) pure substance   c) chemical compound
    b) physical mixture   d) element _____

11. A blended mixture of two or more solids, liquids, or gases is a/an:
    a) solution   c) emulsion
    b) suspension   d) chemical compound _____

12. Liquids that can be mixed together in any proportion without separating are:
    a) suspended   c) emulsified
    b) immiscible   d) miscible _____

13. A substance that dissolves another substance to form a solution, with no change in chemical composition, is a/an:
    a) surfactant   c) emulsion
    b) solvent   d) solute _____

14. A mixture that must be shaken or mixed well before using is a/an:
    a) suspension   c) oil-in-water emulsion
    b) solution   d) water-in-oil emulsion _____

15. Most of the emulsions used in a salon:
    a) are water-in-oil emulsions   c) contain more oil than water
    b) do not use surfactants   d) are oil-in-water emulsions _____

16. Emulsions are mixtures of two or more:
    a) miscible substances   c) immiscible substances
    b) surfactants   d) solutions _____

17. The head of a surfactant molecule is water-loving, or:
   a) immiscible
   c) hydrophobic
   b) hydrophilic
   d) lipophilic
   _____

18. Substances that are often used instead of ammonia in hair products because their odor is not as strong are:
   a) silicone
   c) alkanolamines
   b) alcohol
   d) glycerin
   _____

19. A colorless gas with a strong odor, composed of hydrogen and nitrogen, is:
   a) glycerin
   c) ammonia
   b) fatty alcohol
   d) hydrogen peroxide
   _____

20. In pure water, some of the molecules naturally ionize into hydrogen ions and:
   a) nitrogen ions
   c) hydroxide ions
   b) peroxide ions
   d) oxygen ions
   _____

21. pH is only possible because of the ionization of:
   a) alcohol
   c) oil
   b) water
   d) nonaqueous solutions
   _____

22. The pH scale measures:
   a) acidity and alkalinity
   c) purity and hardness
   b) melting point and boiling point
   d) weight and density
   _____

23. Solutions with a pH below 7.0 are:
   a) neutral
   c) basic
   b) alkaline
   d) acidic
   _____

24. Alkalis have a pH above 7.0 and:
   a) taste sour
   c) soften and swell the hair
   b) turn blue litmus paper red
   d) contract and harden the hair
   _____

25. The average pH of hair and skin is:
   a) seven
   c) three
   b) five
   d) 12
   _____

26. When a substance is combined with oxygen, the process is called:
    a) oxidation
    b) redox reaction
    c) reduction
    d) ionization
    _____

27. The chemical reaction in which hydrogen is added to a substance is:
    a) oxidation
    b) redox reaction
    c) reduction
    d) ionization
    _____

28. A substance that readily transmits electricity is a/an:
    a) insulator
    b) rectifier
    c) converter
    d) conductor
    _____

29. Rubber and silk are good:
    a) insulators
    b) circuit breakers
    c) converters
    d) conductors
    _____

30. A constant electrical current traveling in one direction only is called a/an:
    a) alternating current
    b) direct current
    c) faradic current
    d) sinusoidal current
    _____

31. A unit of electrical pressure is referred to as a/an:
    a) volt
    b) ohm
    c) watt
    d) ampere
    _____

32. An ampere (amp) is a unit of electrical:
    a) strength
    b) tension
    c) resistance
    d) usage
    _____

33. The amount of electrical energy that is being used in one second is measured in:
    a) watts
    b) amps
    c) volts
    d) ohms
    _____

34. A device that automatically interrupts or shuts off an electric circuit in the event of overload is the:
    a) fuse
    b) wall plate
    c) circuit breaker
    d) converter
    _____

35. Electronic facial treatments are known as:
    a) electrotherapy   c) hydrotherapy
    b) light therapy   d) shock therapy   _____

36. The positive electrode of an electrotherapy device is called a/an:
    a) plug   c) wall plate
    b) anode   d) cathode   _____

37. In electrotheraphy, the cathode is:
    a) usually red   c) the positive electrode
    b) the negative electrode d) marked with a plus (+) _____
                                  sign

38. A constant and direct current used to produce chemical effects on the tissues and fluids of the body is the:
    a) sinusoidal current   c) galvanic current
    b) faradic current   d) Tesla current   _____

39. An alternating and interrupted current used to cause muscular contractions is the:
    a) galvanic current   c) faradic current
    b) high-frequency current d) Tesla current   _____

40. An electrical current used for its heat-producing effects is the:
    a) sinusoidal current   c) faradic current
    b) galvanic current   d) high-frequency current _____

41. The anode (positive electrode) of a galvanic device:
    a) expands blood vessels   c) contracts blood vessels
    b) opens the pores   d) produces alkaline   _____
                                  reactions

42. The cathode (negative electrode) of a galvanic device:
    a) soothes nerves   c) stimulates the nerves
    b) closes the pores   d) hardens and firms tissues _____

43. The process of softening and emulsifying oil deposits and blackheads in the follicles is:
    a) cataphoresis   c) desincrustation
    b) anaphoresis   d) iontophoresis   _____

44. Visible light makes up __% of natural sunlight.
    a) 50   c) 35
    b) 5   d) 65   _____

45. Ultraviolet (UV) rays, also called cold rays or actinic rays, have short wavelengths and:
    a) are the least penetrating   c) are safe in large doses
       rays
    b) produce the most heat   d) have no germicidal effect   _____

46. The invisible rays that produce the most heat are the:
    a) ultraviolet rays   c) red light rays
    b) infrared rays   d) actinic rays   _____

47. It is estimated that __ Americans will develop skin cancer.
    a) 1 in five   c) 1 in 1,000
    b) 1 in 100   d) 1 in 50   _____

48. "Combination light" is also known as:
    a) white light   c) ultraviolet light
    b) blue light   d) red light   _____

49. The average distance you should place an infrared lamp from the skin is about:
    a) 18"   c) 30"
    b) 10"   d) 24"   _____

50. A safety precaution you should always follow with electrical equipment is to:
    a) step on electrical cords   c) handle equipment with
                                      wet hands
    b) use only one plug per   d) clean outlets with   _____
       outlet   equipment plugged in

Properties of the Hair and Scalp

1. The scientific study of the hair, its diseases, and its care is called:
   a) dermatology
   b) biology
   c) trichology
   d) hairology
   _____

2. The two main divisions of the hair are the hair root and the:
   a) hair shaft
   b) dermal papilla
   c) bulb
   d) follicle
   _____

3. The three main structures associated with the hair root are the follicle, the bulb, and the:
   a) cuticle
   b) medulla
   c) hair stream
   d) dermal papilla
   _____

4. The hair root is contained in a tube-like depression, or pocket, in the skin known as the:
   a) arrector pili
   b) hair bulb
   c) follicle
   d) sweat pore
   _____

5. The club-shaped structure that forms the lower part of the hair root is the:
   a) hair shaft
   b) dermal papilla
   c) arrector pili
   d) hair bulb
   _____

6. The blood and nerve supply that provides nutrients needed for hair growth are contained in the:
   a) arrector pili
   b) dermal papilla
   c) sebaceous glands
   d) hair shaft
   _____

7. The tiny involuntary muscle in the skin that contracts and causes "goose bumps" is the:
   a) orbicularis oculi
   b) dermal papilla
   c) medulla
   d) arrector pili
   _____

8. The oily substance called sebum is secreted by the:
   a) sudoriferous glands
   b) arrector pili
   c) sebaceous glands
   d) dermal papilla
   _____

9. The three layers of the hair shaft are the cuticle, cortex, and:
   a) follicle
   b) bulb
   c) root
   d) medulla
   _____

10. The layer of the hair shaft that protects it from penetration and damage is the:
    a) cortex
    b) follicle
    c) cuticle
    d) medulla
    _____

11. Generally, only thick, coarse hair contains a:
    a) dermal papilla
    b) cortex
    c) cuticle
    d) medulla
    _____

12. About 90% of the total weight of hair comes from the:
    a) cuticle
    b) medulla
    c) follicle
    d) cortex
    _____

13. Liquids can penetrate the hair only when the __ is raised.
    a) root
    b) medulla
    c) cuticle
    d) cortex
    _____

14. In order to penetrate the cuticle layer and reach the cortex, oxidation haircolors, perm solutions, and chemical relaxers must have:
    a) no pH
    b) an alkaline pH
    c) an acidic pH
    d) a neutral pH
    _____

15. The changes that take place in the hair during permanent waving, chemical relaxing, and oxidation haircoloring occur in the:
    a) medulla
    b) roots
    c) cuticle
    d) cortex
    _____

16. As living cells of the hair mature, they fill up with a protein
    called:
    a) sebum   c) melanin
    b) keratin   d) lanugo   _____

17. The elements that make up the amino acids in hair are
    carbon, nitrogen, hydrogen,:
    a) sulfur and chlorine   c) oxygen and sulfur
    b) copper and oxygen   d) oxygen and sodium   _____

18. Of the five elements in human hair, the element that makes
    up the highest percentage is:
    a) oxygen   c) hydrogen
    b) sulfur   d) carbon   _____

19. The chemical bonds that join amino acids to each other are
    called:
    a) peptide bonds   c) hydrogen bonds
    b) side bonds   d) salt bonds   _____

20. The bonds that account for the strength and elasticity of hair
    are the:
    a) side bonds   c) polypeptide chains
    b) peptide bonds   d) end bonds   _____

21. There are three different types of side bonds in the cortex:
    a) polypeptide, hydrogen, and c) hydrogen, salt, and
       salt bonds   disulfide bonds
    b) salt, hydrogen, and peptide d) disulfide, bisulfide, and   _____
       bonds   salt bonds

22. The strongest side bonds in the cortex are the:
    a) hydrogen bonds   c) salt bonds
    b) peptide bonds   d) disulfide bonds   _____

23. A disulfide bond joins the __ atoms of two neighboring
    cysteine amino acids to create cystine.
    a) carbon   c) nitrogen
    b) hydrogen   d) sulfur   _____

24. Disulfide bonds can be broken by:
    a) shampoo   c) perms and relaxers
    b) heat   d) water   _____

25. A hydrogen bond is a physical side bond that is easily broken by:
    a) changes in pH   c) water or heat
    b) permanent waves   d) chemical relaxers   _____

26. All natural hair color is based on the ratio of:
    a) eumelanin to melanin   c) melanin to aniline
    b) eumelanin to pheomelanin   d) keratin to melanin   _____

27. The pigment that provides natural hair colors from red and ginger to yellow/blonde is:
    a) eumelanin   c) melanin
    b) red melanin   d) pheomelanin   _____

28. All natural hair color is the result of the pigment located within the:
    a) cuticle   c) cortex
    b) pith   d) medulla   _____

29. The amount of movement in the hair strand is referred to as its:
    a) wave pattern   c) texture
    b) density   d) porosity   _____

30. A cross-section of a wavy hair strand is usually:
    a) oval   c) triangular
    b) shapeless   d) round   _____

31. Extremely curly hair that forms coils usually:
    a) is very elastic   c) is very strong
    b) has a coarse texture   d) has a fine texture   _____

32. The four most important factors to consider in a hair analysis include all the following except:
    a) elasticity   c) length
    b) porosity   d) texture   _____

33. Hair texture is defined as the hair's:
    a) ability to absorb moisture   c) ability to stretch
    b) degree of straightness or   d) diameter
       curliness   _____

34. The hair's ability to absorb moisture is its:
    a) porosity   c) elasticity
    b) texture   d) density   _____

35. __ hair has the largest diameter.
    a) fine   c) straight
    b) coarse   d) gray   _____

36. The hair texture that is most susceptible to damage from
    chemical services is:
    a) fine   c) coarse
    b) medium   d) curly   _____

37. The number of individual hair strands on 1 square inch of
    scalp is referred to as:
    a) density   c) porosity
    b) texture   d) coarseness   _____

38. The number of hairs on the head generally varies with the:
    a) percentage of gray   c) color of the hair
    b) texture of the hair   d) person's ethnic
                                        background   _____

39. The thickest hair (highest density) is generally found among
    people with:
    a) black hair   c) red hair
    b) blonde hair   d) brown hair   _____

40. Hair with low porosity is considered:
    a) normal   c) resistant
    b) overly porous   d) ideal   _____

41. Hair with high porosity is generally the result of:
    a) brushing hair before   c) overprocessing
       shampooing
    b) strand testing   d) conditioning treatments _____

42. Wet hair with normal elasticity will stretch up to __ of its original length and return to that same length without breaking.
a) 10%   c) 50%
b) 100%   d) 25%   _____

43. Hair flowing in the same direction is called a:
a) whorl   c) follicle stream
b) hair stream   d) cowlick   _____

44. Dry hair and scalp are caused by:
a) overactive sebaceous glands   c) overproduction of sebum
b) chemical services   d) inactive sebaceous glands   _____

45. All the following characteristics apply to vellus hair except:
a) more abundant on men   c) lacking a medulla
b) found on infants   d) not pigmented   _____

46. Hormonal changes during puberty cause some areas of vellus hair to be replaced with:
a) lanugo   c) gray hair
b) terminal hair   d) medullas   _____

47. The three phases of hair growth are anagen, catagen, and:
a) growth phase   c) transition
b) biogen   d) telogen   _____

48. The growth phase of the hair growth cycle is known as:
a) anagen   c) catagen
b) telogen   d) transition   _____

49. The follicle canal shrinks and detaches from the dermal papilla during the:
a) telogen phase   c) catagen phase
b) anagen phase   d) final phase   _____

50. About __ of scalp hair is growing in the anagen phase at any one time.
a) 90%   c) 1%
b) 10%   d) 50%   _____

51. The phase of hair growth that lasts the shortest time is the:
    a) telogen phase   c) anagen phase
    b) catagen phase   d) dormant phase   _____

52. The resting phase of the hair growth cycle is known as:
    a) catagen   c) telogen
    b) biogen   d) anagen   _____

53. About __ of the hair is in the resting phase at any one time.
    a) 50%   c) 90%
    b) 75%   d) 10%   _____

54. One common hair myth is:
    a) keratin is protein   c) the medulla may be
                                 absent in fine hair
    b) scalp massage increases hair d) hair is shed daily   _____
       growth

55. Gray hair is exactly the same as pigmented hair except that it:
    a) lacks melanin   c) is coarser
    b) is more resistant   d) lacks strength   _____

56. A loss of 35 to 40 hairs a day is considered:
    a) dangerous   c) abnormal
    b) normal   d) unusual   _____

57. Abnormal hair loss is called:
    a) hypertrichosis   c) alopecia
    b) trichoptilosis   d) canities   _____

58. A client's hair must be _____ before any service.
    a) thoroughly dried   c) analyzed
    b) disinfected   d) shampooed   _____

59. By age 35, almost __ percent of men and women show some
    degree of hair loss.
    a) 40   c) 95
    b) 10   d) 25   _____

60. In men, a horseshoe-shaped fringe of hair is referred to as:
    a) horseshoe baldness   c) dome baldness
    b) fringe pattern baldness   d) male pattern baldness   _____

61. A miniaturization of terminal hair contributes to:
    a) canities   c) alopecia areata
    b) androgenic alopecia   d) postpartum alopecia   _____

62. A type of alopecia characterized by the sudden falling out of
    hair in round patches or baldness in spots is called:
    a) androgenic alopecia   c) postpartum alopecia
    b) alopecia areata   d) canities   _____

63. In women, androgenic alopecia shows up as:
    a) general thinning of crown   c) receding front hairline
       hair
    b) gradual loss of side hair   d) hair loss over the entire _____
                                      head

64. Hair loss at the conclusion of a pregnancy is called:
    a) alopecia totalis   c) alopecia areata
    b) postpartum alopecia   d) androgenic alopecia   _____

65. A topical medication applied to the scalp that has been
    proven to stimulate hair growth is:
    a) alum   c) finasteride
    b) follicidil   d) minoxidil   _____

66. Of the two products proven to stimulate hair growth, the oral
    prescription drug is called:
    a) alum   c) sodium hypochlorite
    b) minoxidil   d) finasteride   _____

67. Finasteride is not prescribed for women because of the strong
    potential for:
    a) birth defects   c) excessive hair loss
    b) excessive weight loss   d) excessive hair growth   _____

68. Among the various treatments for hair loss, hair plugs are the:
    a) topical treatment   c) nonmedical treatment
    b) surgical treatment   d) oral treatment   _____

69. Hair plugs may be transplanted by:
    a) cosmetologists   c) surgeons
    b) estheticians   d) barbers   _____

70. The technical term for gray hair is:
    a) alopecia areata   c) canities
    b) pityriasis   d) fragilitas crinium   _____

71. The type of canities that exists at or before birth is known as:
    a) common canities   c) congenital canities
    b) infant canities   d) acquired canities   _____

72. The type of canities that develops with age and is the result
    of genetics is called:
    a) adult-onset canities c) acquired canities
    b) congenital canities   d) common canities   _____

73. Ringed hair is a variety of:
    a) tinea capitis   c) alopecia
    b) canities   d) hypertrichosis   _____

74. The technical term for beaded hair is:
    a) hypertrichosis   c) trichoptilosis
    b) pityriasis   d) monilethrix   _____

75. The technical term for split ends is:
    a) trichoptilosis   c) tinea
    b) canities   d) fragilitas crinium   _____

76. Abnormal growth of hair is called:
    a) pityriasis   c) trichoptilosis
    b) alopecia   d) hypertrichosis   _____

77. A condition characterized by brittleness and nodular swellings
    along the hair shaft is:
    a) trichoptilosis   c) tinea capitis
    b) monilethrix   d) trichorrhexis nodosa   _____

78. Wax hair removal, tweezing, shaving, and electrolysis are among the treatments for:
   a) androgenic alopecia
   b) pityriasis capitis simplex
   c) hypertrichosis
   d) trichorrhexis nodosa   _____

79. The condition in which the hairs may split at any part of their length is called:
   a) pityriasis
   b) trichoptilosis
   c) monilethrix
   d) fragilitas crinium   _____

80. Dry dandruff, thin scales, and an itchy scalp are typical of:
   a) tinea capitis
   b) pityriasis capitis simplex
   c) pediculosis capitis
   d) pityriasis steatoides   _____

81. Pityriasis steatoides is a scalp inflammation marked by:
   a) dry dandruff
   b) greasy or waxy dandruff
   c) red papules
   d) sulfur-yellow, cuplike crusts   _____

82. Clients with tinea capitis should be:
   a) referred to a physician
   b) referred to an esthetician
   c) sanitized and disinfected
   d) treated in the salon   _____

83. Tinea, or ringworm, is caused by:
   a) staphylococci
   b) vegetable parasites
   c) head lice
   d) itch mites   _____

84. Ringworm of the scalp is also known by the technical term:
   a) scutula
   b) tinea capitis
   c) pediculosis capitis
   d) tinea pedis   _____

85. Dry, sulfur-yellow, cuplike crusts on the scalp, called scutula, are characteristic of:
   a) tinea capitis
   b) tinea favosa
   c) pityriasis steatoides
   d) pityriasis capitis simplex   _____

86. The contagious skin disease caused by the itch mite burrowing under the skin is known as:
   a) pediculosis capitis
   b) scabies
   c) carbuncles
   d) tinea favosa   _____

87. Pediculosis capitis is the infestation of the hair and scalp with:
    a) fleas
    b) itch mites
    c) head lice
    d) fungi   _____

88. A boil is also known as:
    a) ringworm
    b) tinea
    c) a furuncle
    d) scabies itch   _____

89. An inflammation of the subcutaneous tissue caused by
    staphylococci is called:
    a) trichoptilosis
    b) dry dandruff
    c) pediculosis capitis
    d) a carbuncle   _____

90. Preventing the spread of tinea, pityriasis, and staphylococci
    infections involves proper:
    a) sanitation and disinfection
    b) medications
    c) inoculation (vaccination)
    d) sterilization   _____

Principles of Hair Design

1. Designing the right hairstyle for your client begins with:
   - a) asking a coworker
   - b) finding a model the client likes
   - c) analyzing the whole person
   - d) looking through style magazines   _____

2. An important factor in being a good hair designer is:
   - a) a strong visual sense
   - b) a pleasing personality
   - c) good conversational skill
   - d) good dexterity   _____

3. Once you have a strong foundation in both technique and styling skills, you can:
   - a) select your clients
   - b) take calculated risks
   - c) rest on your accomplishments
   - d) do only your favorite hairstyles   _____

4. The element of form describes:
   - a) horizontal lines
   - b) overall outline of a hairstyle
   - c) dimension of a style
   - d) wave pattern   _____

5. The term space in hair design refers to:
   - a) proportion
   - b) volume
   - c) line
   - d) the diagonal   _____

6. The use of curved lines in a hair design can be used to:
   - a) emphasize good features
   - b) cover up a bad cut
   - c) create width
   - d) soften a design   _____

7. The use of repeating lines, whether straight or curved:
   a) creates a hard edge
   b) creates more interest in the design
   c) becomes confusing
   d) creates a long, narrow look

   _____

8. Through the use of color in hair design, you can create:
   a) the illusion of more or less volume
   b) a fringe
   c) unusual wave patterns
   d) a slow rhythm pattern

   _____

9. When choosing a new haircolor, one of the considerations is:
   a) the cost of the haircolor
   b) the client's skin tone
   c) the client's wardrobe
   d) facial type

   _____

10. The terms straight, wavy, and curly describe:
    a) wave pattern
    b) rhythm
    c) balance
    d) emphasis

    _____

11. Wave patterns can be altered by the use of:
    a) shampoo
    b) coloring processes
    c) reconditioning treatments
    d) chemicals

    _____

12. One of the principles of hair design, proportion, refers to the:
    a) symmetry
    b) recurrent pattern of movement
    c) relationship between hair, face, and body type
    d) horizontal lines

    _____

13. Using asymmetrical hair design is effective in:
    a) styling fine, straight hair
    b) increasing volume
    c) balancing a large body type
    d) balancing facial features

    _____

14. Ornamentation is an exciting method of creating:
    a) emphasis
    b) rhythm
    c) repeating lines
    d) new wave patterns

    _____

15. A harmonious style creates a look that is:
    a) trendy
    b) proportionate
    c) simple
    d) ornate

    _____

16. When you analyze your client's features, you can style your design to:
    a) disguise hair texture
    b) create more height
    c) play up strengths and minimize weaknesses
    d) emphasize facial type   _____

17. Fine, medium and coarse are qualities that refer to:
    a) proportion
    b) hair texture
    c) concave form
    d) wave pattern   _____

18. Fine, straight hair creates a silhouette that is:
    a) somewhat full
    b) appropriate for everyone
    c) concave
    d) small and narrow   _____

19. The most versatile hair type for styling is:
    a) curly, coarse
    b) curly, fine
    c) straight, medium
    d) wavy, medium   _____

20. If not properly shaped, a very wide silhouette could appear with hair that is:
    a) medium and straight
    b) wavy and fine
    c) wavy and coarse
    d) fine and straight   _____

21. Straight coarse hair has some volume but is:
    a) hard to curl
    b) very fragile
    c) prone to separating
    d) fly-away   _____

22. In hair that is too long, separation can occur and reveal too much scalp if the hair is:
    a) extremely curly and medium
    b) curly and fine
    c) wavy and medium
    d) fine and straight   _____

23. The widest silhouette is found in:
    a) extremely curly, coarse hair
    b) straight, medium hair
    c) wavy, fine hair
    d) curly, medium hair   _____

24. Facial shape is determined by the:
    a) position and prominence of facial bones
    b) measurements
    c) forehead proportion
    d) hairline   _____

25. The generally recognized ideal facial type is considered to be:
    a) convex   c) diamond
    b) oblong   d) oval   _____

26. For design purposes, the three zones of the face are forehead
    to eyebrows, end of the nose to bottom of the chin, and:
    a) ear to ear   c) eyebrows to end of nose
    b) forehead to end of nose   d) nose to upper lip   _____

27. Among the facial shapes is:
    a) trapezoid   c) voluminous
    b) fine   d) inverted triangle   _____

28. If your client has a narrow forehead, it is recommended that
    you:
    a) use bangs   c) direct hair forward over
                                     the sides of the forehead
    b) create a center part   d) style hair away from the   _____
                                     forehead

29. When styling for a client with a long jaw, the hair should be:
    a) full and falls below the jaw   c) symmetrically balanced
    b) cropped to ear length   d) off the face   _____

30. A profile is the outline of a face or figure as seen in a:
    a) front view   c) photograph
    b) mirror   d) side view   _____

31. There are three basic profile types: straight, convex, and:
    a) concave   c) asymmetrical
    b) prominent   d) concise   _____

32. If your client has a convex profile, the hair in the chin area
    should:
    a) hang straight   c) curl tightly
    b) move upward   d) move forward   _____

33. When styling for a client with a large forehead:
    a) use bangs with lots of   c) sweep hair off the face
       volume
    b) use bangs with no volume   d) bring softness to the chin _____
                                     line

34. If your client has a large chin, be sure the hair is:
    a) above or below the chin line
    c) cut straight at the chin line
    b) directed forward in the chin area
    d) at the chin line   _____

35. When a client wears glasses, it will affect how you design the hair:
    a) around the ears
    c) at the chin line
    b) on the forehead
    d) at the nape   _____

36. The three basic parts for bangs are triangular, curved, and:
    a) concave
    c) transitional
    b) diagonal
    d) zigzag   _____

37. The use of a side part helps to:
    a) lessen volume
    c) balance an asymmetrical face
    b) create a dramatic effect
    d) develop height on top   _____

38. When consulting with a male client, recommend styles that are:
    a) not too feminine
    c) short
    b) conservative
    d) flattering and appropriate   _____

39. You can camouflage a receding chin in a male client, with:
    a) a clean-shaven look
    c) longer hair
    b) sideburns
    d) a full beard and mustache   _____

40. A balding male client may look good with a:
    a) closely groomed beard and mustache
    c) bushy sideburns
    b) full beard and mustache
    d) side part   _____

Shampooing, Rinsing, and Conditioning

1. The primary purpose of shampooing in the salon is to:
   a) sell products
   b) wet the hair prior to a service
   c) help the client relax
   d) cleanse the hair and scalp _____

2. When selecting a shampoo, consider the:
   a) humectant in the shampoo
   b) height of the sink
   c) price and profit
   d) condition of the client's hair _____

3. The pH level is an indicator of:
   a) sedimentation
   b) filtration level
   c) oxygen levels
   d) whether a solution is acid or alkaline _____

4. Jheri Redding was the first in the salon industry to market "pH-balanced shampoos," which were:
   a) basic
   b) neutral
   c) more acidic
   d) more alkaline _____

5. Fresh water is purified by:
   a) sedimentation and filtration
   b) water softeners
   c) adding minerals
   d) adding chemicals _____

6. The softness or hardness of water is related to the:
   a) volume
   b) source of the water
   c) weight of the water
   d) amount of minerals present _____

7. The main ingredient of shampoo is:
   a) moisturizers
   b) purified water
   c) surfactant
   d) hard water   _____

8. The effectiveness of surfactants is due to:
   a) the surfactant molecule
   b) vitamin additives
   c) ammonia compounds
   d) protein-based ingredients   _____

9. Surfactant molecules work by:
   a) lifting off oils and dirt into the water
   b) raising the pH of the hair
   c) separating oil and water
   d) deionizing water   _____

10. The highest dollar expenditure for hair care products is for:
    a) shampoo
    b) setting gels
    c) conditioners
    d) haircolor   _____

11. The pH in acid-balanced shampoo is:
    a) the same as in pure water
    b) as high as possible
    c) the same as in chemical treatments
    d) between 4.5 and 5.5   _____

12. Conditioning shampoos contain agents that restore moisture and elasticity and:
    a) relieve scalp conditions
    b) cut through buildup
    c) strip artificial color
    d) add volume   _____

13. Medicated shampoos can be very strong and in some cases:
    a) pick up dirt and oil as you brush through
    b) increase shine
    c) improve manageability
    d) must sit on the scalp for a longer period   _____

14. Clarifying shampoos contain acidic ingredients that:
    a) reduce dandruff
    b) decrease shine
    c) are always a good idea
    d) cut through product buildup   _____

15. Dry shampooing is recommended:
    a) to make hair shiny
    b) for elderly clients
    c) before chemical treatments
    d) to repair damaged hair   _____

16. A shampoo that combines a surfactant base with basic colors is:
    a) therapeutic shampoo
    b) medicated shampoo
    c) acid-balanced shampoo
    d) color-enhancing shampoo _____

17. A temporary remedy for hair that is dry or damaged is:
    a) medicated shampoo
    b) conditioner
    c) dry shampoo
    d) color-enhancing shampoo _____

18. The texture and structure of the hair are controlled by:
    a) chemical processes
    b) heredity, health, and diet
    c) conditioners
    d) scalp conditioners _____

19. Rinse-through finishing rinses are useful for:
    a) deep conditioning
    b) improving the quality of new hair growth
    c) protection against breakage
    d) detangling hair after washing _____

20. For repair and treatment, deep, penetrating conditioners must be left on the hair for:
    a) 30-40 minutes
    b) 10-20 minutes
    c) several hours
    d) 5-10 minutes _____

21. Most conditioners contain:
    a) humectants
    b) hydrophilic molecules
    c) citric acid
    d) surfactants _____

22. The cuticle of the hair is the outermost layer and is made up of:
    a) protective oils
    b) overlapping scales
    c) long strands
    d) melanin scales _____

23. Instant conditioners fall in the pH range of 3.5 to 6.0 and are used to:
    a) restore pH balance
    b) remove oil accumulation from the scalp
    c) add a slight amount of color
    d) improve the condition of the scalp _____

24. Scalp astringent lotion is a conditioning agent applied to the scalp to:
    a) remove oil accumulation   c) soften the scalp
    b) promote healing   d) moisturize the scalp   _____

25. Quaternary ammonium compounds are included in the formulas of moisturizers for their ability to:
    a) attach to hair fibers   c) promote healing of the
                                     scalp
    b) detangle the hair   d) penetrate the cortex   _____

26. To increase hair diameter slightly, choose a:
    a) protein conditioner   c) stiff hairbrush
    b) detanglers   d) cream rinse   _____

27. Concentrated protein conditioners are designed to:
    a) make a bad haircut look   c) penetrate the cortex
       good
    b) eliminate unwanted color d) improve the quality of _____
       tones   new growth

28. Hair treated with a concentrated protein conditioner has all the following qualities except:
    a) equalized porosity   c) improved appearance
    b) improved quality of new   d) increased elasticity   _____
       hair growth

29. Deep conditioning treatments are the chosen therapy when __ is needed.
    a) scalp conditioning   c) equal moisturizing and
                                     protein treatment
    b) thermal protection   d) hair detangling   _____

30. To protect hair from the harmful effects of blow-drying and electric rollers, use:
    a) spray-on thermal protectors c) protein treatment
    b) scalp conditioners   d) hair masks   _____

31. If your client has a dry scalp, the condition may be helped by a:
    a) hair mask   c) protein treatment
    b) detangler   d) scalp conditioner   _____

32. For a client with straight, fine hair, all the following products are recommended except:
   a) volumizing shampoo
   b) moisturizing shampoo
   c) protein treatments
   d) detangler _____

33. If your client has dry, damaged hair, all the following products are recommended except:
   a) gentle cleansing shampoo
   b) spray-on thermal protection
   c) light leave-in conditioner
   d) acid-balanced shampoo _____

34. Correct hair brushing stimulates blood circulation to the scalp and helps:
   a) massage the scalp
   b) remove tangles
   c) loosen scales from the scalp
   d) remove dust, dirt, and spray buildup _____

35. Brushing should be part of most hair services except before a:
   a) chemical service
   b) scalp treatment
   c) scalp massage
   d) shampoo _____

36. The most highly recommended hairbrushes are made from:
   a) wire with rubber tips
   b) natural bristles
   c) widely spaced bristles
   d) nylon bristles _____

37. The best method for hair brushing is to:
   a) brush random areas
   b) part it into sections
   c) brush the scalp vigorously
   d) focus on the ends _____

38. One method of providing scalp stimulation is:
   a) mud pack
   b) scalp conditioner
   c) vigorous combing
   d) massage _____

39. Scalp massage is an extra that keeps your clients coming back, and to be successful it's important to:
   a) have strong hands
   b) know the location of blood vessels
   c) have medical training
   d) do it once or twice a year _____

40. Scalp manipulation techniques include all the following except:
    a) sliding and rotating movement
    b) rapid eye movement
    c) spine movement
    d) relaxing movement   _____

41. The most important rule regarding posture when shampooing is to:
    a) allow your abdomen to relax
    b) lean over the client
    c) keep your shoulders back
    d) round the back   _____

42. All the following items are routinely used when giving a shampoo except:
    a) an infrared lamp
    b) comb and hairbrush
    c) shampoo cape
    d) towels   _____

43. Part of shampoo preparation is to:
    a) apply a scalp steamer
    b) examine the client's hair and scalp
    c) apply an infrared lamp
    d) brush the hair for 15 minutes   _____

44. When performing the shampoo service, an important consideration is:
    a) the water temperature
    b) the nerve points in the neck
    c) the cost of the shampoo
    d) a cold rinse   _____

45. During a shampoo, when manipulating the scalp, use firm pressure if:
    a) the client's scalp is tender
    b) you are performing a chemical service
    c) the client asks for less pressure
    d) the client has healthy hair and scalp   _____

46. After applying small quantities of shampoo, the next step in the shampoo procedure is to:
    a) manipulate the scalp
    b) adjust volume of water
    c) rinse thoroughly
    d) squeeze excess water from hair   _____

47. Part of the cleanup and sanitation process at the end of shampooing is:
   a) scrubbing the entire area
   b) mopping the floor
   c) disinfecting combs and brushes
   d) boiling all combs and brushes   _____

48. Following shampooing and rinsing, the next step is to:
   a) analyze the condition of the hair and scalp
   b) do a thorough brushing
   c) apply a conditioner
   d) do a scalp massage   _____

49. After applying conditioner:
   a) gently comb it through the hair
   b) immediately rinse out
   c) the hair is ready for styling
   d) comb through with a fine-tooth comb   _____

50. When applying a deep conditioning treatment, you may have to:
   a) immediately rinse out
   b) wrap the client in heated towels
   c) place the client under a heated dryer
   d) keep the client in a reclining position   _____

51. After shampooing, chemically treated hair tends to:
   a) be stronger
   b) be oily
   c) tangle
   d) have no body   _____

52. Begin with a shampoo, brushing, and scalp massage when you are doing:
   a) highlighting
   b) chemical relaxing
   c) hairstyling
   d) single-process haircoloring   _____

53. When using dry shampoo for a client with a health problem, apply it:
   a) directly onto the hair
   b) at the ends
   c) only on the scalp
   d) before combing through   _____

54. When servicing clients with special needs, always:
    a) use dry shampoo
    b) shampoo at the bowl
    c) request they shampoo at home
    d) ask their preferences _____

55. The purpose of a general scalp treatment is:
    a) performing a scalp examination
    b) removing oil from the scalp
    c) healing scalp disease
    d) keeping the scalp clean and healthy _____

56. All the following are steps in a normal hair and scalp treatment except:
    a) applying an infrared lamp
    b) vigorously brushing the scalp
    c) brushing the hair for five minutes
    d) applying scalp conditioner _____

57. A dry hair and scalp treatment is recommended for:
    a) a deficiency of natural oil
    b) normal hair
    c) an accumulation of sebum
    d) scalp disease _____

58. A useful appliance for a dry hair and scalp treatment is:
    a) a scalp steamer
    b) a curling iron
    c) a blow-dryer
    d) an infrared lamp _____

59. Kneading the scalp to increase blood circulation is helpful to:
    a) treat scalp disease
    b) treat a dandruff condition
    c) normalize overactive sebaceous glands
    d) balance a deficiency of sebum _____

60. During a dandruff treatment, an effective therapy is:
    a) a deep conditioning treatment
    b) a scalp steamer
    c) chemical relaxers
    d) high-frequency current _____

Haircutting

1. In a haircut, design lines that are proportionate are established by using:
   a) reference points
   b) angles of elevation
   c) cutting lines
   d) subsections
   _____

2. The highest point on the top of the head is called the:
   a) apex
   b) occipital bone
   c) crown
   d) parietal ridge
   _____

3. The widest area of the head, also called the crest area, is the:
   a) occipital bone
   b) four corners
   c) parietal ridge
   d) crown
   _____

4. The bone that protrudes at the base of the skull is the:
   a) hyoid bone
   b) occipital bone
   c) apex
   d) parietal bone
   _____

5. The two front corners represent the widest points in the:
   a) crown area
   b) fringe (bangs) area
   c) apex area
   d) nape area
   _____

6. The area between the apex and the back of the parietal ridge is the:
   a) top
   b) crown
   c) front
   d) sides
   _____

7. The fringe (bangs) area, when combed into natural falling position, falls no farther than:
   a) the outer corners of the nose
   b) behind the ears
   c) the top of the ears
   d) the outer corners of the eyes _____

8. You can locate the top of the head by parting the hair:
   a) at the parietal ridge
   b) down the middle
   c) from ear to ear
   d) at the occipital bone _____

9. Straight lines that are parallel to the horizon, or the floor, are called:
   a) vertical lines
   b) angled lines
   c) horizontal lines
   d) diagonal lines _____

10. The technique in which the ends of the hair are cut at a slight taper, using diagonal lines, is called:
    a) sectioning
    b) blunt cutting
    c) carving
    d) beveling _____

11. The uniform working areas into which the hair is parted for control are called:
    a) angles
    b) elevations
    c) guidelines
    d) sections _____

12. The angle or degree at which a subsection of hair is held from the head when cutting is called:
    a) overdirection
    b) graduation
    c) parting
    d) elevation _____

13. When you elevate the hair below 90 degrees, you are:
    a) creating curl
    b) layering the hair
    c) building weight
    d) removing weight _____

14. As a rule, the more you elevate the hair, the __ you create.
    a) more graduation
    b) more sections
    c) less graduation
    d) less tension _____

15. The section of hair that determines the length the hair will be cut is called the:
    a) elevation
    b) parting
    c) cutting line
    d) guideline _____

16. A guideline that does not move as the haircut progresses is called a:
    a) traveling guideline
    b) interior guideline
    c) first guideline
    d) stationary guideline _____

17. A guideline that moves with you as you work through the haircut is a:
    a) traveling guideline
    b) interior guideline
    c) outline guide
    d) stationary guideline _____

18. The cutting line is the angle at which the:
    a) hair is sectioned
    b) hair is held from the head
    c) traveling guideline moves
    d) fingers are held during cutting _____

19. Combing the hair away from its natural falling position, rather than straight out from the head, toward a guideline is called:
    a) low elevation
    b) 90-degree elevation
    c) overdirection
    d) 45-degree elevation _____

20. When you use overdirection to create a length or weight increase in a haircut, you use a:
    a) traveling guideline
    b) movable guideline
    c) weight line
    d) stationary guideline _____

21. When you are creating __, you use a traveling guide, with no overdirection, to create the same length throughout the haircut.
    a) long layers
    b) a blunt cut
    c) a graduated cut
    d) uniform layers _____

22. Straight hair shrinks when it dries by about:
    a) 1/4 to 1/2 inch
    b) 1/2 inch to two inches
    c) 1/2 to one inch
    d) 1/8 to 1/4 inch _____

23. As it dries, curly hair shrinks by:
    a) 1/2 inch to two inches   c) 1/4 to 1/2 inch
    b) 1/8 to 1/4 inch   d) 1/2 to one inch   _____

24. The direction in which the hair grows from the scalp is called its:
    a) growth pattern   c) wave pattern
    b) hair direction   d) falling pattern   _____

25. An important part of the client consultation before a haircut is analyzing the:
    a) hair color   c) eye color
    b) face shape   d) skin tones   _____

26. The five characteristics that determine the behavior of the hair are: density, texture, wave patterns,:
    a) hairlines and growth   c) hair length and color
       patterns
    b) hair color and growth   d) hairlines and hair length   _____
       patterns

27. Hair texture is based on the:
    a) elasticity of the hair   c) condition of the hair
    b) diameter of each hair   d) amount of curl in the hair   _____
       strand

28. Wave pattern is defined as the amount of __ in the hair strand.
    a) elasticity   c) texture
    b) movement   d) length   _____

29. The tool used to cut blunt or straight lines in the hair is:
    a) a straight razor   c) a clipper
    b) thinning shears   d) haircutting shears   _____

30. When a softer effect is desired on the ends of the hair, the tool generally used is the:
    a) thinning shears   c) a straight razor
    b) an edger   d) haircutting shears   _____

31. The comb generally used in the shears-over-comb technique is the:
    a) barber comb
    b) styling comb
    c) wide-tooth comb
    d) cutting comb _____

32. The tool used mainly to remove bulk from the hair is the:
    a) thinning shears
    b) haircutting shears
    c) clippers
    d) straight razor _____

33. In general, the hand that does most of the work in haircutting is the:
    a) holding hand
    b) nondominant hand
    c) weaker hand
    d) cutting hand _____

34. When holding the shears, the ring finger is placed in the:
    a) finger brace
    b) tang
    c) finger grip of moving blade
    d) finger grip of still blade _____

35. When combing the hair during a haircut, it is necessary to:
    a) palm the shears
    b) hold the comb in the nondominant hand
    c) put the comb down while cutting
    d) put the shears down while combing _____

36. When holding a razor with the handle higher than the shank, the little finger is placed in the:
    a) handle
    b) thumb grip
    c) tang
    d) shank _____

37. The fine teeth of the styling comb are used to:
    a) comb and part the hair
    b) detangle wet hair
    c) comb the subsection before cutting
    d) hold the hair at high elevations _____

38. The amount of pressure applied when combing and holding a subsection of hair is called:
    a) palming
    b) tension
    c) stress
    d) elevation _____

39. A layered haircut can be created with:
    a) traveling guide
    b) stationary guide
    c) transitional line
    d) both a and b _____

40. When cutting uniform or increasing layers, the hand position used most often is:
    a) cutting below the fingers
    b) cutting on the inside of the knuckles
    c) cutting palm to palm
    d) cutting over the fingers _____

41. When cutting with a vertical or diagonal cutting line, the best way to control the subsection is by:
    a) cutting palm to palm
    b) cutting over the palm
    c) cutting on top of the knuckles
    d) cutting over the fingers _____

42. A good safety and sanitation measure is to sweep up cut hair and dispose of it:
    a) before blow-drying the client
    b) after blow-drying the client
    c) as you cut the hair
    d) after the client has left _____

43. The blade in your razor should be replaced:
    a) at the end of the day
    b) at least once a week
    c) prior to each new client
    d) when it's dull or rusty _____

44. The blunt haircut is also referred to as the:
    a) 45-degree cut
    b) 90-degree cut
    c) 180-degree cut
    d) zero-elevation cut _____

45. The graduated haircut is most commonly cut with an elevation of:
    a) 0 degrees
    b) 90 degrees
    c) 180 degrees
    d) 45 degrees _____

46. A long layered haircut is cut at a:
    a) 45-degree angle
    b) 90-degree angle
    c) 180-degree angle
    d) 0-degree angle _____

47. In a layered haircut, the ends of the hair appear:
    a) farther apart
    b) graduated
    c) all one length
    d) closer together _____

48. Cutting hair that is partly damp and partly dry will give you:
   a) an even line
   b) predictable results
   c) uneven results
   d) consistent results

   _____

49. Checking the length of a haircut by parting the hair in the opposite way from which you cut it is called:
   a) palming the shears
   b) cutting palm-to-palm
   c) cross-checking
   d) sectioning

   _____

50. If you use vertical partings in a haircut, you should cross-check the lengths with:
   a) all three partings
   b) vertical partings
   c) horizontal partings
   d) diagonal partings

   _____

51. Tilting the client's head forward while cutting a blunt haircut will result in:
   a) slight graduation of the line
   b) a straight, even line
   c) a layered look
   d) a jagged edge

   _____

52. A classic A-line bob is cut with a:
   a) high elevation
   b) diagonal cutting line
   c) vertical cutting line
   d) 90-degree elevation

   _____

53. In a uniform-layered haircut, all the hair is:
   a) cut at the same length
   b) cut with a perimeter guideline
   c) elevated to 180 degrees
   d) elevated to 45 degrees

   _____

54. Curly hair behaves differently from straight hair; for instance, it:
   a) should only be cut dry
   b) does not expand as much
   c) layers itself naturally
   d) shrinks more after it dries

   _____

55. When cutting curly hair, one tool you should avoid using is:
   a) a styling comb
   b) shears
   c) clippers
   d) a razor

   _____

56. The fringe area is approximately between the:
    a) inner corners of the eyes   c) fronts of the ears
    b) peaks of the eyebrows   d) outer corners of the eyes   _____

57. Cutting the hair with a razor generally gives a softer
    appearance to the hair, in part because the hair ends are cut:
    a) at an angle   c) in jagged lines
    b) below the fingers   d) straight across   _____

58. One way in which razor cutting differs from cutting with
    shears is that:
    a) the guide is above the   c) diagonal lines cannot be
       fingers   cut
    b) the guide is below the   d) only horizontal lines can   _____
       fingers   be cut

59. A razor should not be used on:
    a) dry hair   c) straight hair
    b) wet hair   d) fine hair   _____

60. The method of cutting hair in which the fingers and shears
    glide along the edge of the hair to remove length is called:
    a) point cutting   c) shears-over-comb
    b) slide cutting   d) notching   _____

61. Snipping out pieces of hair at random intervals with the tips
    of the shears is known as:
    a) slide cutting   c) slithering
    b) free-hand notching   d) carving   _____

62. A barbering technique that has crossed over into cosmetology
    is:
    a) carving   c) shears-over-comb
    b) free-hand notching   d) slide cutting   _____

63. When using the shears-over-comb technique, the comb is
    held:
    a) perpendicular to the shears   c) perpendicular to the head
    b) at an angle to the head   d) flush against the head   _____

64. When using the shears-over-comb technique, work with areas:
   a) no wider than the comb
   b) no wider than the blade
   c) as wide as the comb
   d) at least as wide as the blade
   _____

65. In the shears-over-comb technique, an important point to remember is that:
   a) one blade is perpendicular to the comb
   b) both blades keep moving
   c) one blade stays still
   d) the thumb blade is parallel to the comb
   _____

66. The process of removing excess bulk without shortening the length is called:
   a) elevating
   b) texturizing
   c) overdirection
   d) trimming
   _____

67. A texturizing technique similar to razor-over-comb is:
   a) slide cutting
   b) free-hand slicing
   c) razor rotation
   d) free-hand notching
   _____

68. A more modern term for "thinning" is:
   a) removing weight
   b) removing texture
   c) removing curl
   d) removing length
   _____

69. Among the tools to have on hand when clipper cutting, the tool that allows you to cut all the hair evenly to one exact length is the:
   a) thinning shears
   b) haircutting shears
   c) length guard attachment
   d) edger or trimmer
   _____

70. The best way to create a flat-top or square shape close to the scalp is with:
   a) haircutting shears
   b) a razor
   c) clippers
   d) texturizing shears
   _____

71. In the clipper-over-comb technique, the clippers move:
   a) from the bottom to the top of the comb
   b) across the hair above the comb
   c) sideways across the comb
   d) from the top to the bottom of the comb
   _____

72. When cutting with clippers, especially in the nape, always
    work:
    a) with large sections   c) with wet hair
    b) in the direction of natural   d) against the natural   _____
       growth patterns   growth patterns

73. Smaller-sized, cordless clippers used mainly to clean necklines
    and around the ears are called:
    a) tapers   c) edgers
    b) thinners   d) guards   _____

74. The comb used with clippers that allows you to cut the hair
    very short and close to the head is the:
    a) barber comb   c) styling comb
    b) regular cutting comb   d) wide-toothed comb   _____

75. Facial hair is very:
    a) thin   c) soft
    b) coarse   d) fine   _____

Hairstyling

1. The process of shaping and directing the hair into a pattern of S-shaped waves with the fingers, combs, and waving lotion is called:
   a) finger waving
   b) wet setting
   c) thermal curling
   d) thermal waving   _____

2. Waving lotion is a type of hair gel used during finger waving to keep the hair:
   a) wet
   b) dry
   c) pliable
   d) stiff   _____

3. A good waving lotion for finger waving is harmless to the hair and:
   a) should be used liberally
   b) dries on contact
   c) leaves a mild residue
   d) does not flake when dry   _____

4. Finger wave lotion should be applied:
   a) while wearing gloves
   b) to one side of the head at a time
   c) to the entire head after shampooing
   d) with a brush   _____

5. When finger waving, pinching or pushing ridges with the fingers will create:
   a) overdirection of the ridge
   b) inconsistent waves
   c) splits
   d) underdirection of the ridge   _____

6. The three main parts of a pin curl are the base, stem, and:
   a) curl
   b) medulla
   c) wave
   d) circle   _____

7. The section of the pin curl between the base and the first arc is the:
   a) stem
   b) curl
   c) circle
   d) wave _____

8. The stationary part of the pin curl is the:
   a) circle
   b) curl
   c) base
   d) stem _____

9. A tight, firm, long-lasting curl is produced by the:
   a) full-stem curl
   b) mobile stem curl
   c) half-stem curl
   d) no-stem curl _____

10. The greatest curl mobility is achieved with the:
    a) no-stem curl
    b) quarter-turn curl
    c) full-stem curl
    d) half-stem curl _____

11. A section of hair that is molded in a circular movement in preparation for the formation of curls is a:
    a) shaping
    b) parting
    c) base
    d) section _____

12. Open center curls produce:
    a) waves that decrease in size
    b) uniform curls
    c) volume
    d) curls that decrease in size _____

13. Pin curls that are good for fine hair and produce a fluffy curl are:
    a) clockwise pin curls
    b) counterclockwise pin curls
    c) closed center curls
    d) open center curls _____

14. The most common pin curl base you will use is the:
    a) rectangular base
    b) square base
    c) triangular base
    d) arc base _____

15. In a pin curl set, the finished curl is not affected by the:
    a) size of the curl
    b) direction of curl
    c) shape of the base
    d) amount of hair used _____

16. Triangular pin curl bases are used to:
    a) add height
    b) avoid tangling
    c) maintain a smooth upsweep look
    d) prevent splits in the finished style   _____

17. Pin curl bases suitable for curly hairstyles without much volume or lift are the:
    a) arc bases
    b) square bases
    c) rectangular bases
    d) circular bases   _____

18. An important technique to use when making pin curls is:
    a) ribboning
    b) pulling
    c) shaping
    d) squeezing   _____

19. Pin curls sliced from a shaping and formed without lifting the hair from the head are called:
    a) barrel curls
    b) flat curls
    c) cascade or stand-up curls
    d) carved curls   _____

20. Pin curls are correctly anchored when:
    a) they have closed centers
    b) the clip covers the circle
    c) the clip enters at the open end
    d) two clips are used   _____

21. Curls used to create a wave behind a ridge are called:
    a) skip waves
    b) ridge curls
    c) finger waves
    d) clockwise waves   _____

22. Two rows of ridge curls create:
    a) soft curls
    b) maximum height
    c) a strong wave pattern
    d) soft lines between waves   _____

23. Pin curls used to achieve height in the hair design are:
    a) cascade curls
    b) skip waves
    c) ridge curls
    d) carved curls   _____

24. Barrel curls are fastened to the head in a standing position on a:
    a) arc base
    b) rectangular base
    c) circular base
    d) triangular base   _____

25. A roller holds the equivalent of:
    a) 1/2 of a stand-up curl   c) two to four stand-up curls
    b) five stand-up curls   d) one stand-up curl   _____

26. Rollers are different from pin curls in several ways, one way
    being that they:
    a) offer fewer creative   c) take longer to form
       possibilities
    b) work the hair without   d) give a stronger set   _____
       tension

27. The panel of hair on which the roller is placed is called the:
    a) stem   c) circle
    b) base   d) curl   _____

28. The hair between the scalp and the first turn of the roller is
    the:
    a) circle   c) curl
    b) base   d) stem   _____

29. The part of a roller curl that determines the size of the wave
    or curl is the:
    a) base   c) circle or curl
    b) stem   d) clip   _____

30. If hair is wound 1-1/2 turns around a roller, it will create:
    a) a well-anchored curl   c) a C-shape
    b) curls   d) a wave   _____

31. A C shape will result if the hair is wound around the roller:
    a) 1-1/2 turns   c) 2-1/2 turns
    b) one turn   d) five turns   _____

32. The volume achieved in a hairstyle is determined by the size
    of the roller and:
    a) how it sits on its base   c) the direction of the curl
    b) the number of rollers used   d) the anchoring clips used   _____

33. An on-base roller curl produces:
    a) a crisp curl   c) medium volume
    b) the least amount of volume   d) full volume   _____

34. For the least amount of volume in a roller set, use the:
    a) open-end method   c) half-base method
    b) off-base method   d) on-base method   _____

35. A loose roller that is not properly secured to the head will result in:
    a) a longer-lasting set   c) broken hair
    b) larger curls   d) a weak set   _____

36. Hot rollers and Velcro rollers are used:
    a) for minimum volume   c) only on dry hair
    b) only on wet hair   d) for 30 minutes at a time   _____

37. Back-combing and back-brushing are used to:
    a) remove roller indentations   c) keep the hair close to the head
    b) relax the set   d) decrease volume   _____

38. Teasing, ratting, matting, and French lacing are other terms for:
    a) smoothing   c) comb-out
    b) back-brushing   d) back-combing   _____

39. Ruffing is another name for:
    a) smoothing   c) back-brushing
    b) relaxing the set   d) back-combing   _____

40. A technique used to keep curly or extremely curly hair smooth and straight is:
    a) hair wrapping   c) finger waving
    b) wet setting   d) French lacing   _____

41. The part of a blow-dryer that directs the air stream to any section of the hair more intensely is the:
    a) diffuser   c) comb or pick
    b) concentrator   d) fan   _____

42. The diffuser attachment of a blow-dryer causes the air to flow:
    a) in all directions   c) more softly
    b) at a cooler temperature d) at a hotter temperature   _____

43. It is particularly important that the air intake at the back of a blow-dryer be kept:
    a) clear
    b) covered
    c) clogged
    d) cool _____

44. Combs with closely spaced teeth:
    a) shape larger sections of hair
    b) create more surface texture
    c) create a smooth surface
    d) lift the hair away from the head _____

45. A classic styling brush has a:
    a) half-rounded rubber base
    b) ventilated base
    c) generally oval base
    d) large, flat base _____

46. The brush that is generally oval with pure natural bristles or quills of bristle and nylon mix is the:
    a) paddle brush
    b) teasing brush
    c) grooming brush
    d) vent brush _____

47. Smaller round brushes used during blow-drying:
    a) straighten the hair
    b) lift the hair at the scalp
    c) bevel the hair ends
    d) add more curl _____

48. A light, airy, whipped styling product that resembles shaving foam is:
    a) gel
    b) wax
    c) mousse
    d) liquid gel _____

49. The most widely used hairstyling product is:
    a) hair spray
    b) foam or mousse
    c) liquid gel
    d) pomade _____

50. A hairstyling product that adds considerable weight to the hair is:
    a) foam or mousse
    b) pomade or wax
    c) liquid gel
    d) silicone shiner _____

51. Guidelines for blow-drying the hair include directing the blow-dryer:
    a) toward the scalp
    b) against direction in which hair is wound
    c) at one section until dry
    d) from scalp to ends _____

52. Creating an updo can be difficult on hair that has been:
    a) blow-dried
    b) freshly washed
    c) set in hot rollers
    d) pressed
    _____

53. Another term for thermal waving is:
    a) hair pressing
    b) Grateau waving
    c) marcel waving
    d) ironing the hair
    _____

54. Thermal waving and curling are done on:
    a) wet hair
    b) unwashed hair
    c) towel-dried hair
    d) dry hair
    _____

55. To hold an even temperature, thermal irons should be made of the best quality:
    a) zinc
    b) steel
    c) magnesium
    d) hard rubber
    _____

56. A conventional thermal iron is:
    a) coal-heated
    b) electric self-heated, vaporizing
    c) electric self-heated
    d) stove-heated
    _____

57. Electric vaporizing irons should not be used on pressed hair because they cause the hair to:
    a) return to its natural curly state
    b) become flat and limp
    c) become straighter
    d) weaken and break
    _____

58. For white, lightened, or tinted hair, it is advisable:
    a) to use large thermal irons
    b) to use hot thermal irons
    c) not to use thermal irons
    d) to use lukewarm thermal irons
    _____

59. The styling portion of a thermal iron consists of a rod and:
    a) shell
    b) prong
    c) cord
    d) swivel
    _____

60. The required temperature of heated thermal irons depends on the:
    a) cosmetologist's speed
    b) texture of the hair
    c) type of irons selected
    d) size of the heater
    _____

61. The temperature of heated thermal irons is tested on:
    a) wax paper
    b) a damp cloth
    c) a strand of hair
    d) a piece of tissue paper   _____

62. A thermal comb should be made of:
    a) steel
    b) hard rubber
    c) wood
    d) plastic   _____

63. When manipulating thermal irons, the rolling movement should be done with the:
    a) fingers
    b) hand
    c) wrist
    d) arm   _____

64. To give a finished appearance to hair ends, use:
    a) spiral curls
    b) end curls
    c) the figure 8 technique
    d) the figure 6 technique   _____

65. A method of thermal-curling the hair by winding a strand around the rod to create hanging curls is:
    a) volume thermal iron curls
    b) end curls
    c) the figure 6 technique
    d) spiral curls   _____

66. Volume thermal iron curls are used to provide a finished hairstyle with:
    a) tension
    b) lift
    c) separation
    d) depth   _____

67. A volume-base thermal curl is formed by placing the curl:
    a) completely off its base
    b) in the center of its base
    c) forward and high on its base
    d) half off its base   _____

68. Full-base thermal curls provide:
    a) maximum lift or volume
    b) a strong curl with moderate volume
    c) slight lift or volume
    d) a strong curl with full volume   _____

69. In half-base curls the hair is held at a:
    a) 125-degree angle
    b) 70-degree angle
    c) 90-degree angle
    d) 135-degree angle   _____

70. The thermal curl that offers the least lift or volume is the:
    a) volume-base curl
    c) half-base curl
    b) off-base curl
    d) full-base curl _____

71. To ensure a good thermal curl or wave, the hair must be:
    a) damp
    c) clean
    b) prepared with setting lotion d) well oiled _____

72. In thermal curling or waving, fishhook hair ends are caused when the:
    a) hair ends protrude from the c) curl is started too high
       irons
    b) curl is started too low
    d) irons are too hot _____

73. Hair pressing:
    a) temporarily curls straight c) permanently waves hair
       hair
    b) temporarily straightens hair d) gives wide waves to curly _____
       hair

74. Hair straightening, or pressing, is a popular service that lasts:
    a) until the next shampoo
    c) from haircut to haircut
    b) until the next day
    d) one week _____

75. Types of hair pressing are the soft press, hard press, and:
    a) figure 8 press
    c) light press
    b) croquignole press
    d) medium press _____

76. The type of hair pressing that removes 50% to 60% of the curl is the:
    a) soft press
    c) hard press
    b) minimum press
    d) medium press _____

77. The temperature of the pressing comb should be adjusted to the hair's:
    a) length
    c) texture
    b) cleanliness
    d) style _____

78. The least difficult type of hair to press is:
    a) medium curly hair
    c) resistant, curly hair
    b) wiry, curly hair
    d) virgin hair _____

79. The type of hair that requires the least heat and pressure with a pressing comb is:
a) medium   c) coarse
b) short   d) fine   _____

80. Applying a heated pressing comb twice on each side of the hair is known as a:
a) soft press   c) regular press
b) hard press   d) comb press   _____

81. Burnt hair strands:
a) seal in the hair oil   c) cannot be conditioned
b) help hold certain styles d) only occur in a hard press   _____

82. In pressing coarse hair, more heat is required because it:
a) has an enlarged cuticle   c) contains a medulla
b) is never gray   d) has the greatest diameter   _____

83. To avoid breakage when pressing fine hair, you should use:
a) less heat and pressure   c) more heat and pressure
b) no pressing oil   d) more protective cream   _____

84. The use of excess heat on gray, tinted, or lightened hair may:
a) alter future hair growth c) ruin the pressing comb
b) discolor the hair   d) make the hair wiry   _____

85. Failure to correct dry and brittle hair before thermal straightening may result in:
a) overcurling   c) hair breakage
b) a weaker result d) more retouch treatments   _____

86. To avoid smoke or burning while pressing hair, use:
a) more pressing oil   c) more heat
b) preheated pressing oil d) less pressing oil   _____

87. A hard press in which a hot curling iron is passed through the hair first is called:
a) a double press   c) a thermal press
b) a rod press   d) a chemical press   _____

88. Hair pressing treatments between shampoos are called:
    a) light presses
    b) touch-ups
    c) re-presses
    d) soft presses
    _____

89. Hair that is wiry and curly:
    a) is difficult to press
    b) is easiest to press
    c) requires less pressing oil
    d) requires relaxing before pressing
    _____

90. Before performing a hair press, the hair should be divided into:
    a) Nine sections
    b) Three sections
    c) Four sections
    d) Five sections
    _____

91. A scalp may be classified as normal, flexible, or:
    a) thin
    b) tight
    c) brittle
    d) porous
    _____

92. Applying the thermal pressing comb once on each side of the hair is required for a:
    a) soft press
    b) hard press
    c) croquignole press
    d) double press
    _____

93. Pressing combs should be constructed of good-quality steel or:
    a) plastic
    b) hard rubber
    c) brass
    d) zinc
    _____

94. The actual pressing or straightening of the hair is accomplished with the comb's:
    a) tail
    b) back rod
    c) handle
    d) teeth
    _____

95. Pressing oil may be applied either before or after the hair is:
    a) pressed
    b) sectioned
    c) thoroughly dried
    d) shampooed
    _____

96. The hair and scalp may be conditioned with special hair products, hair brushing, and:
    a) intense rinsing
    b) lemon rinses
    c) dry shampoo
    d) scalp massage
    _____

97. The metal portion of a pressing comb may be immersed in a solution of __ for 1 hour to give it a smooth and shiny appearance.
    a) alcohol and shampoo
    b) hot baking soda
    c) ammonia
    d) sodium hypochlorite
    _____

98. Too frequent hair pressing treatments can cause:
    a) breaking and shortening of the hair
    b) excessive oiliness
    c) hirsuties
    d) hypertrichosis
    _____

99. Carbon may be removed from the pressing comb by rubbing with:
    a) pressing oil
    b) disinfectant
    c) a wet towel
    d) fine sandpaper
    _____

100. Do not use __ when pressing short hair at the temples and back of the neck.
    a) moderate heat
    b) high heat
    c) a pressing comb
    d) a temple comb
    _____

Braiding and Braid Extensions

1. The art of braiding, which is an important tradition in many cultures, originated in:
   - a) Africa
   - b) Norway
   - c) India
   - d) Native America   _____

2. In traditional cultures, braiding patterns often signified:
   - a) number of siblings
   - b) literacy
   - c) social and marital status
   - d) manual dexterity   _____

3. Natural hairstyling works with the hair's:
   - a) color
   - b) length
   - c) braids
   - d) curl or coil pattern   _____

4. In the context of braiding, hair texture involves three qualities; wave pattern, feel, and:
   - a) diameter
   - b) length
   - c) symmetry
   - d) chemical history   _____

5. When styling with braids for a round facial type, it is useful to include:
   - a) symmetry
   - b) updo braiding
   - c) fullness at the sides
   - d) dreadlocks   _____

6. The right tools are essential for braiding, including:
   - a) large rollers
   - b) clippers
   - c) a curling iron
   - d) a tail comb   _____

7. The material kanekalon is used for:
   - a) hair treatments
   - b) synthetic hair extensions
   - c) hackles
   - d) drawing boards   _____

8. In general, it is best to braid the hair:
   a) after trimming
   b) when it is damp
   c) when it is dry
   d) without shampooing

   _____

9. Textured hair presents styling challenges because it is:
   a) fragile both wet and dry
   b) limp and lacking body
   c) straight
   d) flyaway

   _____

10. When preparing textured hair for braiding, separate thicker hair into:
    a) few sections
    b) uneven sections
    c) many sections
    d) more sections in front

    _____

11. A three-strand braid created with the underhand technique is called a/an:
    a) invisible braid
    b) rope braid
    c) fishtail braid
    d) visible braid

    _____

12. The overhand pick-up technique is used to create:
    a) an invisible braid
    b) a rope braid
    c) cornrows
    d) box braids

    _____

13. A braid made with two strands twisted around each other is called:
    a) natural hairstyling
    b) dreadlocks
    c) canerows
    d) a rope braid

    _____

14. A fishtail braid is a two-strand braid in which hair is:
    a) twisted to the left
    b) picked up from the sides
    c) rolled in a clockwise direction
    d) braided underhand

    _____

15. Single braids, box braids, and individual braids are all:
    a) underhand stitch braids
    b) cornrows
    c) dreadlocks
    d) free-hanging braids

    _____

16. The partings for single braids can be square, triangular, or:
    a) rectangular
    b) circular
    c) random
    d) arc-shaped

    _____

17. The foundation of beautiful cornrows is:
    a) the comb technique   c) consistent and even
                                partings
    b) layering   d) extensions   _____

18. When using the feed-in method of cornrowing, you are
    adding:
    a) large clips   c) ornamentation
    b) extensions   d) spiral revolutions _____

19. Dreadlocks can be started using the:
    a) flat, contoured style c) on-the-scalp braid
                                technique
    b) brush technique   d) palm roll   _____

20. In the development of dreadlocks, the lock is closed at the
    end and the hair is tightly meshed into a ropelike cylinder
    during the:
    a) atrophy stage   c) maturation stage
    b) sprouting stage   d) growing stage   _____

Wigs and Hair Enhancements

1. In classic body proportions, the ratio of head size to body is about:
   a) 1 to 7
   b) 1 to 10
   c) 1 to 5
   d) 1 to 12 _____

2. During a client consultation for hair enhancements, it is best if the client is in:
   a) a facial bed
   b) a salon smock
   c) a salon cape
   d) her street clothes _____

3. Human hair wigs can be distinguished from synthetic hair wigs by a simple:
   a) strand test
   b) match test
   c) predisposition test
   d) pull test _____

4. The advantages of human hair wigs over synthetic wigs include:
   a) colors that do not oxidize
   b) low cost
   c) unlimited colors
   d) greater durability _____

5. Synthetic wigs have many advantages over human hair wigs, such as:
   a) tolerance for high heat
   b) pre-set cut, color, and texture
   c) a more natural look than human hair
   d) no need for shampooing _____

6. The human hair that is considered top of the line for wigs is:
   a) virgin European hair
   b) Indian hair
   c) color-treated European hair
   d) Asian hair _____

7. An animal hair whose natural white color lends itself to adding fantasy colors is:
   a) goat hair
   c) horse hair
   b) sheep hair
   d) yak hair _____

8. The second most costly hair available for wigs is from:
   a) India and Asia
   c) South America
   b) the U.S.
   d) Europe _____

9. Indian hair is naturally:
   a) straight
   c) wavy
   b) coiled
   d) curly _____

10. Cuticle-intact hair is more expensive because the hair is:
    a) rooted hair
    c) synthetic hair
    b) turned hair
    d) fallen hair _____

11. Cap wigs:
    a) are usually hand-knotted
    c) have an open framework
    b) are made with wefts
    d) are machine-made _____

12. The hair addition that consists of rows of wefts sewn to elastic strips in a circular pattern is a:
    a) sewn extension
    c) capless wig
    b) cap wig
    d) toupee _____

13. Wigs that most closely resemble actual human hair growth are:
    a) integration
    c) machine-made
    b) hand-tied
    d) semi-hand-tied _____

14. Wigs that are a combination of synthetic hair and hand-tied human hair are:
    a) semi-hand-tied wigs
    c) integration wigs
    b) hand-knotted wigs
    d) fused wigs _____

15. The method of wig construction that is the least expensive is the:
    a) hand-tied wig
    c) machine-made wig
    b) semi-hand-tied wig
    d) hand-knotted wig _____

16. Two methods used to prepare the hair for putting on a wig are the hair wrap and:
    a) a French twist
    b) pin curls
    c) roller curls
    d) a ponytail _____

17. When shampooing a wig, you may use a/an:
    a) alkaline shampoo
    b) dandruff shampoo
    c) shampoo with a sulfur base
    d) gentle shampoo _____

18. When you cut and style a wig, the wig should be placed on a block during:
    a) combing out
    b) haircutting
    c) blow-drying
    d) shampooing _____

19. When styling a wig, the aim is to make it look:
    a) plastered down
    b) artificial
    c) realistic
    d) perfect _____

20. If you are going to custom-color a human hair wig, you should use hair that has been:
    a) tinted with metallic dye
    b) colored to level 0
    c) treated with a filler
    d) decolorized or bleached _____

21. If you use an oxidizing haircolor on hair that has been treated with metallic dye, the:
    a) result will look artificial
    b) color will take more effectively
    c) hair will swell and smoke
    d) result will look more natural _____

22. A human hair wig should not be permed if it has been:
    a) treated with metallic dye
    b) colored with semipermanent color
    c) custom-colored with permanent color
    d) lightened _____

23. A hairpiece:
    a) gives 20% to 50% coverage
    b) is permanently attached
    c) is worn during sleep
    d) sits on top of the hair _____

24. A hair addition with an opening in the base through which the client's own hair is pulled to blend with the added hair is called a/an:
    a) integration hairpiece
    b) track-and-sew extension
    c) wig
    d) toupee

    _____

25. Hairpieces particularly suited for men with severe hair loss, but that are also worn by women, are:
    a) integration hairpieces
    b) hair extensions
    c) toupees
    d) wraparound ponytails

    _____

26. Hair extensions are attached to the:
    a) base of the hair
    b) hairline
    c) ends of the hair
    d) scalp

    _____

27. In the track-and-sew method, hair extensions are attached to:
    a) the client's scalp
    b) on-the-scalp braids
    c) a ponytail
    d) off-the-scalp braids

    _____

28. The method of attaching hair wefts or single strands with an adhesive or glue gun is called:
    a) track and sew
    b) fusion
    c) taping
    d) bonding

    _____

29. Before you apply bonded extensions, always perform a:
    a) patch test
    b) temperature test
    c) test curl
    d) strand test

    _____

30. Extension hair is bonded to the client's own hair with material activated by a special heating tool in the method called:
    a) bonding
    b) track and sew
    c) fusion
    d) gluing

    _____

Chemical Texture Services

1. Hair services that cause a chemical change that permanently alters the natural wave pattern of the hair are called:
   a) thermal waving
   b) chemical texture services
   c) wet setting
   d) haircoloring services
   _____

2. A strong, compact cuticle makes for:
   a) damaged hair
   b) easily permed hair
   c) resistant hair
   d) porous hair
   _____

3. Porous, damaged, or chemically treated hair requires a perm solution that is:
   a) high pH
   b) more alkaline
   c) stronger
   d) less alkaline
   _____

4. Changing the natural wave pattern of the hair is made possible by the breaking of the:
   a) side bonds
   b) peptide bonds
   c) end bonds
   d) polypeptide chains
   _____

5. Of the three types of side bonds, disulfide bonds are the:
   a) most easily broken
   b) strongest
   c) weakest
   d) most numerous
   _____

6. Salt bonds are easily broken by:
   a) water
   b) blow-dryers
   c) changes in pH
   d) high humidity
   _____

7. An example of a physical change is a:
   a) chemical relaxing
   b) soft curl permanent
   c) permanent wave
   d) wet set
   _____

8. Hydrogen bonds are very weak, but they account for about __ of the hair's total strength.
   a) 1/2   c) 1/4
   b) 1/3   d) 1/6   _____

9. By making a point of keeping accurate, up-to-date client records, you will:
   a) take longer to perform a   c) improve your technical
      service   skills
   b) annoy the client   d) repeat past mistakes   _____

10. The most important factors to consider in a hair analysis for chemical texture services are texture, density, porosity, elasticity, and:
    a) length   c) color
    b) hairline   d) growth direction   _____

11. Hair texture is described with the terms:
    a) porous and resistant   c) straight, wavy, curly, coiled
    b) coarse, medium, and fine   d) high and low   _____

12. When treated with chemical texture services, coarse hair is usually:
    a) easier to process   c) harder to penetrate
    b) more susceptible to damage   d) more fragile   _____

13. The hair texture that is the most fragile and easiest to process with permanent waving solution is:
    a) fine hair   c) medium hair
    b) porous hair   d) coarse hair   _____

14. The single most important factor in determining the ability of hair to hold a curl is its:
    a) density   c) porosity
    b) elasticity   d) texture   _____

15. Wet hair with normal elasticity can stretch up to __ percent of its original length and then return to that length without breaking.
    a) 50   c) 25
    b) 80   d) 70   _____

16. The first part of any perm, wrapping the hair on perm rods, causes a/an:
    a) disulfide bond change
    b) chemical change
    c) end bond change
    d) physical change
    _____

17. The second part of any perm, the application of waving solution and neutralizer, causes a:
    a) physical change
    b) chemical change
    c) hydrogen bond change
    d) peptide bond change
    _____

18. The major difference between a wet set and a perm is the:
    a) size of the wrapping tools
    b) type of end bonds broken
    c) type of wrapping tool
    d) type of side bonds broken
    _____

19. The size of the perm tool determines the:
    a) base control
    b) placement of the curl
    c) size of the curl
    d) base direction
    _____

20. Wrapping the hair on small tools increases the:
    a) tension
    b) curl size
    c) side bonds broken
    d) hydrogen bonds broken
    _____

21. For perm wrapping, the hair is divided into panels, then into:
    a) partings
    b) base controls
    c) subpanels
    d) base sections
    _____

22. The position of the tool in relation to its base section is called the:
    a) base control
    b) base direction
    c) tool angle
    d) wrapping technique
    _____

23. Base control is determined by the angle:
    a) in which the hair is combed
    b) of the hair to the length of the tool
    c) at which the tool is positioned on the head
    d) at which the hair is wrapped
    _____

24. The hair is wrapped at an angle 45 degrees beyond perpendicular to its base section in:
    a) half-off-base placement
    b) on-base placement
    c) cross-base placement
    d) off-base placement
    _____

25. In off-base placement, the hair is wrapped __ to its base
    section.
    a) 45 degrees above   c) 45 degrees below
       perpendicular   perpendicular
    b) parallel   d) perpendicular (90 degrees) _____

26. Because it places additional stress and tension on the hair,
    caution should be used with:
    a) off-base placement   c) spiral wrapping
    b) croquignole wrapping   d) on-base placement   _____

27. Of the various base controls, the least amount of volume is
    created by using:
    a) off-base placement   c) croquignole placement
    b) on-base placement   d) half-off-base placement   _____

28. The angle at which the perm tool is positioned on the head is
    referred to as the:
    a) base section   c) wrapping technique
    b) base control   d) base direction   _____

29. The wrapping technique in which the hair is wrapped from
    the ends to the scalp in overlapping layers is called:
    a) basic wrapping   c) spiral wrapping
    b) croquignole wrapping   d) circular wrapping   _____

30. In the spiral perm wrapping technique, the hair is wrapped:
    a) in overlapping layers   c) at an angle other than
                                    perpendicular
    b) at a perpendicular angle d) from ends to scalp only   _____

31. Rods with a smaller circumference in the center than at the
    ends are called:
    a) convex rods   c) straight rods
    b) tapered rods   d) concave rods   _____

32. Rods with the same circumference along their entire length or
    curling area are called:
    a) straight rods   c) convex rods
    b) tapered rods   d) concave rods   _____

33. The distinguishing feature of soft bender rods is that they can be:
    a) used with a croquignole wrap
    b) fastened to form a circle
    c) bent into many shapes
    d) used with a spiral wrap _____

34. Circle tools or loop rods are ideal for:
    a) wrapping small sections
    b) croquignole wrapping short hair
    c) wrapping very short hair
    d) spiral wrapping very long hair _____

35. End wraps are absorbent papers used when winding hair on perm tools to:
    a) control the hair ends
    b) absorb moisture
    c) control elasticity
    d) maintain moisture _____

36. When you place one end paper over the top of the hair strand as you wrap it around the perm tool, it is called a:
    a) double flat wrap
    b) single flat wrap
    c) one-way wrap
    d) bookend wrap _____

37. When you fold one end paper in half over the hair ends like an envelope, it is called a:
    a) bookend wrap
    b) double end paper wrap
    c) single end paper wrap
    d) half wrap _____

38. The end paper technique that provides the most control over the hair ends and keeps them evenly distributed is the:
    a) bookend wrap
    b) single flat wrap
    c) convex wrap
    d) double flat wrap _____

39. Permanent waving solution breaks the disulfide bonds in the cortex through a chemical reaction called:
    a) subtraction
    b) hydrogenation
    c) reduction
    d) oxidation _____

40. In permanent waving solutions, thiol compounds act as:
    a) reducing agents
    b) oxidizing agents
    c) neutralizing agents
    d) alkalizing agents _____

41. Ammonium thioglycolate is produced by adding __ to thioglycolic acid.
    a) alcohol
    b) neutralizer
    c) hydrogen peroxide
    d) ammonia   _____

42. Alkaline waves are also called:
    a) acid-balanced waves
    b) low-pH waves
    c) cold waves
    d) ammonia-free waves   _____

43. Most true acid waves:
    a) have a pH between 3 and 5
    b) process quickly
    c) produce a very firm curl
    d) require heat to speed processing   _____

44. Most of the acid waves in today's salons have a pH between:
    a) 6.5 to 7.0
    b) 7.8 and 8.2
    c) 7.0 to 9.6
    d) 4.5 to 7.0   _____

45. Permanent waves that require heat from an outside source, usually a hair dryer, are called:
    a) acid-balanced
    b) alkaline
    c) endothermic
    d) exothermic   _____

46. One benefit of ammonia-free waves is that they:
    a) are good for very resistant hair
    b) have no unpleasant ammonia odor
    c) are less alkaline than ammonia solutions
    d) are less damaging than ammonia solutions   _____

47. In permanent waving, most of the processing takes place as soon as the solution penetrates the hair, within the first:
    a) 5 to 10 minutes
    b) 3 to 5 minutes
    c) 15 to 30 minutes
    d) 10 to 15 minutes   _____

48. Complete saturation of the hair is essential to proper processing in all permanent waves, but especially on:
    a) thick hair
    b) porous hair
    c) fine hair
    d) resistant hair   _____

49. A properly processed permanent wave should break and
rebuild about ___ percent of the hair's disulfide bonds.
    a) 50   c) 75
    b) 90   d) 25   _____

50. If the hair is underprocessed:
    a) too many disulfide bonds   c) the hair is curlier at the
       are broken   scalp
    b) the hair is overly softened d) too few disulfide bonds   _____
                                      are broken

51. Neutralizer performs two functions, deactivating any
remaining waving solution in the hair and:
    a) rebuilding broken disulfide c) re-forming broken
       bonds   hydrogen bonds
    b) conditioning the hair   d) breaking remaining   _____
                                      disulfide bonds

52. The chemical reaction involved in neutralizing is:
    a) hydrogenation   c) oxidation
    b) activating   d) reduction   _____

53. Perm solution should be rinsed from the hair for at least:
    a) three minutes   c) ten minutes
    b) eight minutes   d) five minutes   _____

54. Perm solution should be rinsed from the hair before
neutralizing to avoid scalp irritation and:
    a) underprocessing   c) neutralizing the perm
                                      solution
    b) lightening the hair color   d) darkening the hair color _____

55. After rinsing perm solution from the hair, the next step is to:
    a) remove the rods   c) blot the rods with towels
    b) apply more waving solution d) apply neutralizer   _____

56. An optional step after blotting the hair and before applying
neutralizer is to:
    a) apply a pre-neutralizing   c) rinse a second time
       conditioner
    b) wash with a gentle   d) apply protective cream   _____
       shampoo

57. The hydrogen atoms in the broken disulfide bonds are so strongly attracted to the oxygen in the neutralizer that they release their bond with the:
a) sulfur atoms
b) nitrogen atoms
c) salt bond
d) sodium
_____

58. Unless the scalp is irritated, hair that has just been permed may be colored with:
a) oxidation haircolor
b) demipermanent haircolor
c) a double-process color application
d) permanent haircolor
_____

59. It is safe to perm hair that:
a) has been colored with metallic haircolor
b) has been treated with hydroxide relaxer
c) shows signs of breakage
d) has been treated with thio relaxer
_____

60. Metallic salts leave a coating on the hair that may cause severe discoloration, hair breakage, or:
a) uneven curls
b) mild odor
c) hair straightening
d) smooth curls
_____

61. To test for metallic salts in the hair, immerse at least 20 strands in a mixture of peroxide and:
a) thio
b) bleach
c) alcohol
d) ammonia
_____

62. The basic perm wrap is also called a:
a) bricklay perm wrap
b) weave technique
c) straight set wrap
d) curvature perm wrap
_____

63. The perm wrap that creates a movement that curves within sectioned-out panels is the:
a) weave technique
b) straight perm wrap
c) bricklay perm wrap
d) curvature perm wrap
_____

64. Zigzag partings are used to divide base areas in the perm wrapping technique called the:
a) bricklay perm
b) spiral technique
c) weave technique
d) curvature perm
_____

65. The double tool perm technique is also called the:
    a) curvature wrap
    b) spiral technique
    c) bricklay wrap
    d) piggyback wrap _____

66. The spiral perm technique:
    a) uses two tools on one strand of hair
    b) produces a uniform curl from scalp to ends
    c) follows the curvature of the head
    d) is particularly suited for short hair _____

67. To determine the proper processing time needed for optimal curl development, you should do:
    a) preliminary test curls
    b) a strand test
    c) an elasticity test
    d) a patch test _____

68. When giving a partial perm, you can make a smooth transition from a rolled to an unrolled section by using a __ as the last tool next to an unrolled section.
    a) concave tool
    b) circle tool
    c) pin curl
    d) larger tool _____

69. The process of rearranging the basic structure of extremely curly hair into a straight form is called:
    a) thermal hair relaxing
    b) chemical hair waving
    c) chemical hair relaxing
    d) permanent waving _____

70. Chemical hair relaxing is very similar to:
    a) permanent haircoloring
    b) permanent waving
    c) hair pressing
    d) thermal waving _____

71. All relaxers and permanents change the shape of the hair by:
    a) creating hydrogen bonds
    b) breaking hydrogen bonds
    c) creating disulfide bonds
    d) breaking disulfide bonds _____

72. Most relaxers contain the same ingredients used in:
    a) permanent haircolors
    b) temporary haircolors
    c) depilatories
    d) epilators _____

73. Extremely curly hair:
    a) has a uniform diameter
    b) has varying diameters
    c) is very strong
    d) is thickest at the twists _____

74. Extremely curly hair is weakest at the:
   a) midshaft
   b) base
   c) ends
   d) twists _____

75. Thio relaxers:
   a) have a pH above 10
   b) use less ATG than in perming
   c) harden the hair
   d) do not use a reducing agent _____

76. Each step in the pH scale represents a __ change in concentration.
   a) twofold
   b) twentyfold
   c) hundredfold
   d) tenfold _____

77. Hydroxide relaxers remove one atom of sulfur from a disulfide bond and convert it into a lanthionine bond in a process called:
   a) reduction
   b) neutralization
   c) lanthionization
   d) oxidation _____

78. The disulfide bonds that are broken by hydroxide relaxers:
   a) can never be re-formed
   b) are re-formed by lanthionization
   c) are changed into hydrogen bonds
   d) are re-formed by neutralizer _____

79. The neutralization of hydroxide relaxers involves the use of:
   a) oxidizing neutralizer
   b) acid-balanced shampoo
   c) high-pH shampoo
   d) hydrogen peroxide _____

80. If you have treated a client's hair with a hydroxide relaxer, it cannot be treated with:
   a) future hydroxide relaxers
   b) thermal waving
   c) soft curl permanents
   d) permanent haircolor _____

81. Metal hydroxide relaxers are ionic compounds formed by a metal combined with:
   a) oxygen and nitrogen
   b) nitrogen and hydrogen
   c) hydrogen and sulfur
   d) oxygen and hydrogen _____

82. Sodium hydroxide relaxers are commonly called:
    a) no-lye relaxers
    b) lye relaxers
    c) no-mix no-lye relaxers
    d) low-pH relaxers   _____

83. A chemical relaxer that straightens the hair completely but with much less scalp irritation than other hydroxide relaxers is:
    a) guanidine hydroxide relaxer
    b) sodium hydroxide relaxer
    c) lithium hydroxide relaxer
    d) low-pH relaxer   _____

84. Chemical relaxers marketed as mild alternative relaxers are:
    a) guanidine hydroxide relaxer
    b) sodium hydroxide relaxer
    c) lithium hydroxide relaxer
    d) sulfites   _____

85. Mild strength relaxers are recommended for fine, damaged, or:
    a) medium-curly hair
    b) medium-texture hair
    c) color-treated hair
    d) coarse, extremely curly hair   _____

86. The application for a virgin relaxer begins:
    a) 1/4" to 1/2" away from the scalp
    b) along the entire strand
    c) at the scalp
    d) at the new growth   _____

87. Relaxer should be applied to the most resistant area first, which is usually the:
    a) front hairline
    b) temples
    c) back of the head
    d) nape   _____

88. Normalizing solutions are conditioners with an acidic pH that are used in a relaxing procedure:
    a) prior to shampooing
    b) before applying relaxer
    c) after shampooing
    d) before rinsing out relaxer   _____

89. To determine if the hair is sufficiently relaxed, do:
    a) a patch test
    b) periodic strand testing
    c) a test curl
    d) a porosity test   _____

90. To neutralize hydroxide relaxer, shampoo the hair with an acid-balanced shampoo at least:
    a) three times
    b) once
    c) twice
    d) five times
    _____

91. A soft curl permanent:
    a) relaxes the hair slightly
    b) makes existing curls larger
    c) makes tighter curls
    d) straightens the hair
    _____

92. A Jheri curl or soft curl permanent is a combination of a thio relaxer and:
    a) thermal waving
    b) a hydroxide permanent
    c) a hydroxide relaxer
    d) a thio permanent
    _____

93. In a soft curl permanent, the hair is first relaxed, then wrapped:
    a) on horizontal base sections
    b) on base
    c) off base
    d) on vertical base sections
    _____

94. When applying a hydroxide relaxer:
    a) the client's hair must be damp
    b) gloves are not necessary
    c) begin at the scalp and hair ends
    d) do not shampoo first
    _____

95. You should not attempt to remove more than __ of the natural curl with chemical relaxing.
    a) 50%
    b) 80%
    c) 30%
    d) 70%
    _____

Haircoloring

1. Pure or fundamental colors that cannot be achieved from a
   mixture are called:
   a) tertiary colors   c) complementary colors
   b) secondary colors   d) primary colors   _____

2. A tertiary color is achieved by mixing equal amounts of a
   secondary color and its neighboring:
   a) complementary color   c) cool color
   b) primary color   d) secondary color   _____

3. A primary and secondary color positioned opposite each other
   on the color wheel are:
   a) tertiary colors   c) cool colors
   b) warm colors   d) complementary colors   _____

4. A secondary color is obtained by mixing equal amounts of
   two:
   a) primary colors   c) cool colors
   b) complementary colors   d) tertiary colors   _____

5. Red, yellow, and blue are considered:
   a) secondary colors   c) primary colors
   b) cool colors   d) warm colors   _____

6. The darkest primary color is:
   a) violet   c) red
   b) blue   d) yellow   _____

7. The secondary colors are orange, violet, and:
   a) green   c) blue
   b) yellow   d) white   _____

8. The equal combination of yellow and blue creates:
   a) orange
   b) a tertiary color
   c) a warm color
   d) green
   _____

9. A complementary color combination is:
   a) red and yellow
   b) red and green
   c) red and violet
   d) red and orange
   _____

10. Blue-green and red-violet are:
    a) tertiary colors
    b) neutralizing colors
    c) primary colors
    d) complementary colors
    _____

11. Fine-textured hair:
    a) has an average response to color
    b) is resistant to lightening
    c) may process lighter
    d) takes color faster
    _____

12. The hair texture likely to take longer to process is:
    a) medium hair
    b) thin hair
    c) coarse hair
    d) fine hair
    _____

13. Hair that is resistant and requires a longer processing time usually has:
    a) low porosity
    b) a fine texture
    c) high porosity
    d) average porosity
    _____

14. Hair with high porosity has a:
    a) resistant cuticle
    b) tight cuticle
    c) lifted cuticle
    d) a slightly raised cuticle
    _____

15. If you test the hair between your fingers and it feels smooth, it has:
    a) low elasticity
    b) low porosity
    c) normal elasticity
    d) high porosity
    _____

16. The underlying color that emerges during lightening is known as:
    a) contributing pigment
    b) pheomelanin
    c) eumelanin
    d) intensity
    _____

17. The type of melanin that gives the hair black and brown color is:
    a) pheomelanin
    b) mixed melanin
    c) dark melanin
    d) eumelanin   _____

18. Level is used to identify the:
    a) strength of a color tone
    b) warmth or coolness of a color
    c) lightness or darkness of a color
    d) base color   _____

19. Intensity describes the:
    a) primary and secondary colors
    b) strength of a color tone
    c) lightness or darkness of a color
    d) warmth or coolness of a color   _____

20. A base color is the:
    a) strength of a color tone
    b) pigment under the natural color
    c) lightness or darkness of a color
    d) predominant tonality of a color   _____

21. The warmth or coolness of a color is known as its:
    a) level
    b) depth
    c) tone
    d) intensity   _____

22. Hair lightening is also called bleaching or:
    a) decolorizing
    b) stripping
    c) uncoloring
    d) presoftening   _____

23. Haircolors are divided into four general classifications based on their chemistry, which, in turn, affects the final color result and:
    a) retail price
    b) developer strength
    c) intensity
    d) lasting ability   _____

24. Raising the cuticle of the hair so that the tint can penetrate is the function of the:
    a) developer
    b) tint molecules
    c) alkalizing ingredient
    d) oxidizing agent   _____

25. The function of hydrogen peroxide in haircolor is to:
    a) raise the cuticle
    b) make the developer alkaline
    c) destroy the melanin
    d) break up the melanin   _____

26. Temporary haircolor:
    a) makes a physical change
    b) requires a strand test
    c) lasts 4 to 6 shampoos
    d) penetrates the cortex   _____

27. The pigment molecules of semipermanent haircolor are:
    a) larger than temporary color molecules
    b) only coat the cuticle
    c) smaller than permanent color molecules
    d) smaller than temporary color molecules   _____

28. The haircolor category that is considered semipermanent:
    a) requires a patch test
    b) requires ammonia
    c) penetrates the cortex
    d) lasts 4 to 6 weeks   _____

29. Demipermanent haircolor deposits color but does not:
    a) penetrate the hair shaft
    b) lift color
    c) cover unpigmented hair
    d) require a patch test   _____

30. In recent years, demipermanent haircolor has been used exclusively on the __ of previously colored hair.
    a) new growth
    b) resistant areas
    c) midshaft to ends
    d) base area   _____

31. The only haircolor that has a lifting action on the hair is:
    a) temporary
    b) permanent
    c) semipermanent
    d) demipermanent   _____

32. Permanent haircolors are considered permanent because the tint molecules:
    a) are trapped in the cortex
    b) coat the cortex
    c) are trapped in the cuticle
    d) stain the cuticle   _____

33. Permanent haircolors contain uncolored dye precursors known as:
    a) color fillers
    b) toners
    c) developers
    d) aniline derivatives   _____

34. The agent that, when mixed with an oxidative haircolor, supplies the oxygen to develop color molecules and create a change in hair color is the:
    a) alkalizing agent
    b) developer
    c) aniline derivatives
    d) ammonia

35. The most commonly used oxidizer in haircoloring is:
    a) ammonia
    b) oxygen
    c) aniline
    d) hydrogen peroxide

36. Developers have a pH between:
    a) 4 and 6.5
    b) 10 and 13
    c) 2.5 and 4.5
    d) 8.5 and 10.5

37. The hydrogen peroxide used to provide maximum lift in a one-step color service is:
    a) 10 volume
    b) 30 volume
    c) 20 volume
    d) 40 volume

38. Henna is a type of:
    a) metallic dye
    b) oxidative tint
    c) natural haircolor
    d) semipermanent color

39. Gradual colors, historically marketed to men, are also called:
    a) vegetable haircolors
    b) metallic haircolors
    c) men's haircolors
    d) oxidative tints

40. Lighteners work by:
    a) removing melanin
    b) toning melanin
    c) destroying melanin
    d) dispersing melanin

41. As soon as hydrogen peroxide is mixed into a lightener formula, it begins to:
    a) add hydrogen
    b) release oxygen
    c) darken the melanin
    d) reduce oxygen

42. Toners are used primarily on:
    a) permanently colored hair
    b) glazed hair
    c) prelightened hair
    d) damaged hair

43. When you decolorize a client's hair, your goal is to create the correct degree of:
    a) contributing pigment
    b) porosity
    c) yellow
    d) final color _____

44. The hair should never be lifted with lightener past:
    a) yellow-gold
    b) gold
    c) white
    d) pale yellow _____

45. The most critical part of the color service is the:
    a) processing
    b) comb-out
    c) consultation
    d) rinsing _____

46. A client consultation for haircoloring should include:
    a) examining the client in the mirror
    b) stating the cost of the service
    c) recommending one option
    d) booking an extra 5 minutes _____

47. A release statement is used mainly to explain:
    a) what damages the client may not sue for
    b) your malpractice insurance policy
    c) if hair is in proper condition to receive color
    d) that you cannot be sued for haircolor mistakes _____

48. A predisposition test is performed to determine:
    a) haircolor results
    b) allergy to aniline
    c) proper application method
    d) processing time _____

49. A preliminary strand test should be performed:
    a) if the client requests it
    b) if the hair is to be cut
    c) in the lower crown
    d) at the nape _____

50. Once a temporary color rinse has been applied:
    a) rinse with warm water
    b) apply conditioner
    c) apply a plastic cap
    d) style as desired _____

51. How well semipermanent colors "take" depends on the:
    a) hair's wave pattern
    b) formula strength
    c) hair's porosity
    d) volume of hair _____

52. The application procedure for demipermanent haircolor is similar to that for:
   a) temporary color
   b) foil lightening
   c) permanent color
   d) semipermanent color _____

53. In a double-process color application, the lightener is followed by application of:
   a) color remover
   b) bleach
   c) the depositing color
   d) a presoftener _____

54. Hair at the scalp processes color faster due to:
   a) body heat
   b) incomplete melanin growth
   c) more open cuticle layers
   d) greater porosity _____

55. Overlapping previously colored or lightened hair can:
   a) cause streaking
   b) create lines of demarcation
   c) retard hair growth
   d) irritate the scalp _____

56. Demipermanent color may be applied to hair ends during a retouch procedure only if:
   a) the color is darker
   b) required by the manufacturer
   c) the color is faded
   d) it has been four weeks between retouches _____

57. Oil lightener is used to:
   a) perform a tint back
   b) remove old haircolor
   c) lift four or more levels
   d) lift one or two levels _____

58. Cream lighteners may be mixed with dry crystals known as:
   a) activators
   b) fillers
   c) blonders
   d) color removers _____

59. Off-the-scalp lighteners:
   a) tend to run and drip
   b) are very gentle
   c) come in powder form
   d) are used for retouching _____

60. Powder lighteners should not be used for:
   a) foil lightening
   b) balayage
   c) off-the-scalp lightening
   d) retouch services _____

61. Hair takes longer to lighten:
    a) the stronger the lightener is
    b) the more melanin it has
    c) the less porous it is
    d) the less red there is in the natural color

    _____

62. When heat is used along with lightening chemicals, it softens the hair and can make it:
    a) slower to process
    b) more resistant
    c) stronger
    d) more fragile

    _____

63. If a preliminary strand test for lightening indicates the hair is not light enough, you can:
    a) increase the processing time
    b) recondition the hair
    c) decrease the processing time
    d) decrease the strength of the mixture

    _____

64. Partings for applying lightener should be:
    a) 1"
    b) 1/4"
    c) 1/2"
    d) 1/8"

    _____

65. In a lightening procedure, when you check a strand for lightening, you should:
    a) blow-dry the strand
    b) rub the strand with a damp towel
    c) blot the strand with a damp towel
    d) shampoo the strand

    _____

66. Before using a toner, you must achieve the proper:
    a) level
    b) foundation
    c) texture
    d) tone

    _____

67. There are __ degrees of decolorizing.
    a) 10
    b) 3
    c) 5
    d) 7

    _____

68. When a lightener is applied so that it overlaps previously lightened hair:
    a) a toner is required
    b) the hair may not accept color
    c) a soap cap is required
    d) breakage may occur

    _____

69. Using conditioner on the hair at the end of a toner application:
a) opens the cuticle
b) lowers the pH
c) raises the pH
d) seals the color in _____

70. Coloring some hair strands lighter than the natural color is called:
a) highlighting
b) reverse highlighting
c) lowlighting
d) lightening _____

71. Lowlighting is the technique of coloring strands of hair:
a) to counter brassy tones
b) darker than the natural color
c) lighter than the natural color
d) with red for red highlights _____

72. The degree of highlighting or lowlighting you can achieve with the cap technique depends on the:
a) the size of the hook
b) how large you cut the holes
c) how much lightener you apply
d) number of strands pulled through _____

73. A complete haircolor record should include the:
a) client's signature
b) amount of hair cut
c) client's scalp condition
d) hairstyle desired _____

74. Painting a lightener directly onto clean, styled hair is known as the:
a) cap technique
b) balayage technique
c) reverse highlighting technique
d) foil technique _____

75. If a client has unwanted orange tones, use a haircolor with a:
a) violet base
b) green base
c) blue base
d) yellow base _____

76. Presoftening is performed on gray or resistant hair to:
a) open the cuticle
b) soften melanin
c) create added warmth
d) open the cortex _____

77. Fillers are used to equalize porosity and:
    a) diffuse melanin
    b) deposit a base color
    c) remove color buildup
    d) open the cuticle _____

78. The foil technique of lightening can be done by either weaving or:
    a) hooking
    b) painting
    c) folding
    d) slicing _____

79. Tint removal may be performed if:
    a) the haircolor is too light
    b) the haircolor is too dark
    c) the hair will not absorb toner
    d) lightener did not lift enough _____

80. When performing a tint back:
    a) a filler may be used
    b) a lightener should be used
    c) the hair may need to be cut
    d) the hair should be presoftened _____

81. After a tint has been mixed and used, any leftover tint:
    a) should be tightly sealed
    b) is safe to use for 24 hours
    c) should be discarded
    d) becomes a semipermanent color _____

82. When formulating permanent color for hair that is 10–30% gray, your color choice should be:
    a) 2 parts desired level and 1 part lighter level
    b) the desired level
    c) equal parts desired and lighter level
    d) 1 level lighter _____

83. When selecting a color filler:
    a) reduce the additional primary color
    b) replace the hair's missing primary color
    c) replace the hair's missing secondary color
    d) reduce the additional secondary color _____

84. The first step in properly camouflaging excessive brassiness is to:
   a) identify actual color of brassiness
   b) remove tint with dye remover
   c) perform a patch test
   d) use a violet-based tint _____

85. A soap cap involves using shampoo with:
   a) filler
   b) oil bleach
   c) a color rinse
   d) tint _____

86. A highlighting shampoo is a combination of shampoo and:
   a) a semipermanent tint
   b) hydrogen peroxide
   c) an aniline derivative tint
   d) an oil bleach _____

87. An example of a double-process color application is:
   a) presoftening and tinting
   b) conditioning and toning
   c) shampooing and applying temporary color
   d) shampooing and applying demipermanent color _____

88. A "gun-metal gray" shade is:
   a) a degree of decolorization
   b) a desirable shade of gray
   c) a sign that the hair is overly porous
   d) the color of 50% unpigmented hair _____

89. A glaze, sometimes used to give the hair shine and tone, is usually a/an:
   a) demipermanent color
   b) permanent color
   c) on-the-scalp lightener
   d) temporary color _____

90. Highlighting services are also known as:
   a) temporary lightening
   b) dimensional haircoloring
   c) partial lightening
   d) three-dimensional coloring _____

91. When a very slight change in hair shade is desired, or when the client's hair processes very rapidly, consider using a:
   a) highlighting shampoo tint
   b) highlighting conditioner
   c) permanent haircolor
   d) temporary color rinse _____

Histology of the Skin

1. The study of the skin and its nature, structure, functions, diseases, and treatment is known as:
   a) trichology
   b) dermatology
   c) etiology
   d) pathology
   _____

2. A specialist in the cleansing, preservation of health, and beautification of the skin and body is a/an:
   a) pathologist
   b) trichologist
   c) esthetician
   d) dermatologist
   _____

3. Healthy skin is:
   a) slightly acid
   b) free from bacteria
   c) slightly alkaline
   d) free of sebum
   _____

4. The skin is thinnest on the:
   a) back of the hands
   b) eyelids
   c) eyebrows
   d) forehead
   _____

5. Of all the skin on the body, the thickest is on the:
   a) abdomen
   b) thighs
   c) knees and elbows
   d) palms and soles
   _____

6. The outer protective layer of the skin is called the:
   a) adipose
   b) epidermis
   c) reticular
   d) dermis
   _____

7. The epidermis does not contain any:
   a) blood vessels
   b) keratin
   c) melanocytes
   d) nerve endings
   _____

8. Nerves, hair follicles, papillae, and sweat and oil glands are found in the:
   a) epidermis
   b) scarf skin
   c) subcutaneous tissue
   d) dermis
   _____

9. The stratum corneum has scale-like cells made up of:
   a) melanin
   b) keratin
   c) sebum
   d) elastin
   _____

10. The layer of the epidermis that is continually being shed and replaced is the:
    a) stratum germinativum
    b) stratum lucidum
    c) stratum granulosum
    d) stratum corneum
    _____

11. The stratum corneum is also known as the:
    a) basal layer
    b) horny layer
    c) clear layer
    d) granular layer
    _____

12. The growth of the epidermis begins in the:
    a) stratum corneum
    b) stratum granulosum
    c) stratum germinativum
    d) stratum lucidum
    _____

13. Melanin, which protects sensitive cells from the destructive effects of excessive UV rays, is found in the __ of the epidermis.
    a) stratum granulosum
    b) stratum germinativum
    c) stratum corneum
    d) stratum lucidum
    _____

14. The reticular and papillary layers are found in the:
    a) subcutis
    b) scarf skin
    c) true skin
    d) Malpighian layer
    _____

15. The small, cone-shaped elevations at the bottom of the hair follicles are:
    a) tactile corpuscles
    b) melanocytes
    c) arrector pili
    d) papillae
    _____

16. The layer of the dermis that supplies the skin with oxygen and nutrients is the:
    a) reticular layer
    b) stratum germinativum
    c) papillary layer
    d) derma
    _____

17. Subcutaneous tissue is a:
    a) clear layer
    b) fatty layer
    c) highly sensitive layer
    d) granular layer   _____

18. The skin is nourished by:
    a) sebum
    b) melanin
    c) keratin
    d) blood and lymph   _____

19. Sensory nerve fibers in the skin react to:
    a) light
    b) fear
    c) cold
    d) oil secretion   _____

20. The motor nerve fibers of the skin:
    a) cause goose bumps
    b) excrete perspiration
    c) react to heat
    d) control the flow of sebum   _____

21. The skin gets its strength, form, and flexibility from:
    a) keratin and melanin
    b) blood and lymph
    c) collagen and elastin
    d) sensory and motor nerves   _____

22. A protein fiber that helps the skin regain its shape, even after being repeatedly stretched, is:
    a) sebum
    b) adipose tissue
    c) keratin
    d) elastin   _____

23. The sudoriferous glands regulate:
    a) body temperature
    b) oil flow
    c) excess dryness
    d) emotional response   _____

24. Sebaceous glands are found in all parts of the body except for the:
    a) face and scalp
    b) forehead
    c) palms and soles
    d) eyelids   _____

25. The small openings of the sweat glands on the skin are called:
    a) fundus
    b) follicles
    c) ducts
    d) sweat pores   _____

26. The excretion of sweat from the skin is under the control of the:
    a) circulatory system   c) nervous system
    b) muscular system   d) endocrine system   _____

27. The palms, soles, forehead, and armpits contain particularly numerous:
    a) hair follicles   c) salivary glands
    b) sudoriferous glands   d) sebaceous glands   _____

28. The sebaceous glands secrete:
    a) blackheads   c) oil
    b) salt   d) perspiration   _____

29. The duct of a sebaceous gland opens into the:
    a) hair follicle   c) sweat pore
    b) bloodstream   d) fundus   _____

30. The function of sebum is to:
    a) promote new skin growth   c) excrete perspiration
    b) lubricate the skin   d) minimize calluses   _____

31. The blood and sweat glands of the skin regulate body heat by maintaining a Fahrenheit temperature of about:
    a) 98.6°   c) 86.9°
    b) 93.5°   d) 96.8°   _____

32. Approximately 80 to 85 percent of the skin's aging is caused by:
    a) poor diet   c) the sun's rays
    b) lack of exercise   d) heredity   _____

33. Skin tissues wrinkle and sag because of the weakening of the:
    a) arrector pili muscles   c) layers of the epidermis
    b) collagen and elastin fibers   d) hair follicles   _____

34. The ultraviolet rays of the sun that are also called the "aging rays" are the:
    a) UVB rays   c) UVA rays
    b) visible rays   d) infrared rays   _____

35. The "burning rays" that can damage the skin and eyes are:
    a) infrared rays
    b) UVA rays
    c) blue rays
    d) UVB rays
    _____

36. Ultraviolet exposure is highest between the hours of:
    a) 10 A.M. and 3 P.M.
    b) 8 A.M. and 6 P.M.
    c) 9 A.M. and 1 P.M.
    d) 10 A.M. to 5 P.M.
    _____

37. UVB rays cause tanning of the skin by affecting the:
    a) elastin fibers
    b) melanocytes
    c) collagen fibers
    d) papillae
    _____

38. Nicotine in tobacco causes contraction and weakening of the:
    a) collagen fibers
    b) cranial bones
    c) facial nerves
    d) blood vessels
    _____

39. An excessive intake of alcohol:
    a) contracts blood vessels
    b) creates scar tissue
    c) overdilates blood vessels
    d) draws water to the tissues
    _____

40. If a client has an inflamed skin disorder that is not infectious, you should:
    a) wear gloves
    b) suggest self-treatment
    c) prescribe treatment
    d) refer the client to a physician
    _____

41. A papule is a:
    a) hypertrophy of the skin
    b) primary skin lesion
    c) secondary skin lesion
    d) subjective symptom
    _____

42. Pus is most likely to be found in:
    a) vesicles
    b) macules
    c) pustules
    d) leukoderma
    _____

43. Poison oak and poison ivy produce:
    a) vesicles
    b) wheals
    c) excoriation
    d) papules
    _____

44. The skin lesions found in chapped lips and hands are:
    a) papules
    b) tumors
    c) stains
    d) fissures
    _____

45. A closed, abnormally developed sac containing fluid, semifluid, or morbid matter is a:
    a) cyst
    b) keloid
    c) papule
    d) pustule
    _____

46. After an injury heals, a __ may develop.
    a) furuncle
    b) vesicle
    c) cicatrix
    d) carbuncle
    _____

47. An abnormal cell mass is known as a:
    a) macule
    b) tumor
    c) papule
    d) keloid
    _____

48. Before a wound or blemish has healed completely, it is likely to be covered with a:
    a) scar
    b) cyst
    c) crust
    d) keloid
    _____

49. Dandruff is an example of:
    a) milia
    b) scale
    c) sebaceous gland disorder
    d) fissure
    _____

50. Comedone is the technical name for:
    a) blackhead
    b) macule
    c) nevus
    d) whitehead
    _____

51. Milia is the technical name for:
    a) pimples
    b) nevus
    c) whiteheads
    d) blackheads
    _____

52. Disorders of the sebaceous glands do not include:
    a) miliaria rubra
    b) acne
    c) rosacea
    d) asteatosis
    _____

53. Acne, or common pimples, is also known as acne simplex or:
    a) acne singularis
    b) acne vulgaris
    c) acne rosacea
    d) cystic acne
    _____

54. Rosacea is a chronic congestion on the cheeks and nose characterized by:
    a) fever blisters
    b) dry skin
    c) dilation of blood vessels
    d) inflammation of sweat glands
    _____

55. One of the symptoms of asteatosis is:
    a) fever blisters
    b) dry skin
    c) oily skin
    d) clear blisters
    _____

56. In seborrhea, the appearance of the skin is:
    a) oily and shiny
    b) scaly
    c) red and blotchy
    d) dry and dull
    _____

57. Steatomas usually appear on the:
    a) legs
    b) arms
    c) scalp
    d) face
    _____

58. Bromhidrosis means:
    a) excess sebum
    b) lack of sebum
    c) foul-smelling perspiration
    d) lack of perspiration
    _____

59. Excessive sweating is called:
    a) hyperhidrosis
    b) asteatosis
    c) anhidrosis
    d) bromhidrosis
    _____

60. People exposed to excessive heat may develop a condition known as:
    a) anhidrosis
    b) eczema
    c) bromhidrosis
    d) miliaria rubra
    _____

61. Eczema is an inflammation of the skin characterized by:
    a) fatty tumors
    b) dry or moist lesions
    c) white-silver scales
    d) fever blisters
    _____

62. Red patches covered with silver-white scales may indicate the presence of:
    a) herpes simplex
    b) seborrhea
    c) eczema
    d) psoriasis
    _____

63. Herpes simplex is a recurring:
    a) viral infection
    b) bacterial infection
    c) non-contagious disease
    d) 24-hour virus
    _____

64. Certain chemicals found in cosmetics may cause:
    a) miliaria rubra
    b) dermatitis simplex
    c) occupational simplex
    d) dermatitis venenata
    _____

65. The common term for lentigines is:
    a) calluses
    b) freckles
    c) birthmarks
    d) warts
    _____

66. Albinism is characterized by an:
    a) absence of melanin
    b) excess of melanin
    c) absence of sebum
    d) excess skin growth
    _____

67. Liver spots are technically known as:
    a) leukoderma
    b) chloasma
    c) nevus
    d) plasma
    _____

68. The skin disorder that is further classified as vitiligo and albinism is:
    a) carcinoma
    b) hypertrophy
    c) chloasma
    d) leukoderma
    _____

69. An abnormal skin discoloration that occurs during aging or after certain diseases is known as a:
    a) stain
    b) nevus
    c) lentigo
    d) hypertrophy
    _____

70. A birthmark is also known as a:
    a) stain
    b) nevus
    c) chloasma
    d) leukoderma
    _____

71. Continued pressure or friction on the hands and feet may result in the formation of a:
    a) verruca
    b) tumor
    c) keratoma
    d) nevus
    _____

72. A hypertrophy that occurs most often on the neck of an older person is called a:
a) verruca
b) skin tag
c) keratoma
d) mole
_____

73. A hypertrophy that is caused by a virus and is infectious is the:
a) verruca
b) mole
c) skin tag
d) keratoma
_____

74. The most common and least severe type of skin cancer is:
a) malignant keratoma
b) malignant melanoma
c) basal cell carcinoma
d) leukoderma
_____

75. Black or dark brown patches on the skin that may be uneven in texture, jagged, or raised are characteristic of:
a) malignant melanoma
b) basal cell carcinoma
c) vitiligo
d) herpes simplex
_____

76. A skin cancer characterized by scaly red papules or nodules is:
a) leukoderma
b) malignant melanoma
c) squamous cell carcinoma
d) basal cell carcinoma
_____

77. The vitamin that promotes the production of collagen in the skin is:
a) vitamin E
b) vitamin A
c) vitamin D
d) vitamin C
_____

78. Retinoic acid or Retin-A is the topical form of:
a) vitamin A
b) vitamin E
c) vitamin D
d) vitamin C
_____

79. Vitamin E, when used with vitamin A, helps protect the skin from the harmful effects of:
a) alcohol abuse
b) a poor diet
c) the sun's rays
d) lack of exercise
_____

80. Water composes __ percent of the body's weight.
a) 50 to 70
b) 80 to 90
c) 10 to 20
d) 40 to 50
_____

Hair Removal

1. The growth of an unusual amount of hair on parts of the body normally bearing only downy hair is called:
   - a) monilethrix
   - b) canities
   - c) hirsuties
   - d) trichoptilosis
   _____

2. Electrolysis may be performed only by a/an:
   - a) cosmetologist
   - b) licensed electrologist
   - c) cosmetology instructor
   - d) esthetician
   _____

3. Electrolysis removes hair by means of:
   - a) epilation
   - b) intense light
   - c) a laser beam
   - d) an electric current
   _____

4. In electrolysis, the electric current is applied with a/an:
   - a) laser beam
   - b) electrode
   - c) plug
   - d) light ray
   _____

5. The method of hair removal that uses intense light to destroy the hair follicles is:
   - a) photo-epilation
   - b) laser hair removal
   - c) threading
   - d) electrolysis
   _____

6. Photo-epilation can provide __ percent clearance of hair in 12 weeks.
   - a) 20 to 30
   - b) 90 to 100
   - c) 70 to 80
   - d) 50 to 60
   _____

7. In laser hair removal, a laser beam is used to impair the:
   - a) hair follicles
   - b) nerves
   - c) capillaries
   - d) muscles
   _____

8. The absolute requirement for laser hair removal is that the hair must be:
   a) fine, downy hair
   b) pale blond to white
   c) lighter than the skin
   d) darker than the skin _____

9. The determining factor in whether or not a cosmetologist may perform photo-epilation or laser hair removal on clients is:
   a) state or province law
   b) manufacturer's guidelines
   c) cosmetology school instruction
   d) manufacturer's training _____

10. Shaved hair feels thicker because the:
    a) hair root is enlarged
    b) follicle shrinks
    c) hair ends are blunt
    d) skin is contracted _____

11. When preparing a client with normal skin for shaving, cleanse the face with a:
    a) very wet towel
    b) warm towel
    c) cold towel
    d) hot towel _____

12. To soften the eyebrows prior to tweezing, place cotton pledgets or a towel saturated with __ over the brows.
    a) astringent
    b) alcohol
    c) cold water
    d) warm water _____

13. During eyebrow tweezing, the area should be sponged with cotton moistened with:
    a) disinfecting solution
    b) soapy water
    c) antiseptic lotion
    d) warm water _____

14. After completing a tweezing procedure, sponge the eyebrows and surrounding skin with:
    a) brush sanitizer
    b) warm water
    c) soapy water
    d) astringent _____

15. In electronic tweezing, radio frequency energy is transmitted down the hair shaft and causes dehydration of the:
    a) dermis
    b) papilla
    c) epidermis
    d) nerve _____

16. The method of removing superfluous hair by dissolving it at the skin level makes use of a/an:
    a) epilator
    c) laser beam
    b) cotton thread
    d) depilatory
    _____

17. When a depilatory is applied, the hair expands and the:
    a) cuticle is stripped away
    c) disulfide bonds break
    b) texture changes
    d) polypeptide bonds break
    _____

18. An epilator removes superfluous hair by:
    a) pulling it out of the follicle
    c) destroying the hair root
    b) dissolving it at skin level
    d) impairing the follicles
    _____

19. The time between waxings is generally:
    a) 1 to 2 weeks
    c) 3 to 4 months
    b) 4 to 6 weeks
    d) 4 to 6 months
    _____

20. For waxing to be effective, the length of the hair should be at least:
    a) ¼ to ½ inch
    c) ⅛ to ¼ inch
    b) ½ to 1 inch
    d) 1 to 1-½ inch
    _____

21. The temperature of hot wax should be tested on:
    a) your fingertip
    c) your wrist
    b) the client's wrist
    d) wax paper
    _____

22. In a hot waxing treatment, the wax should be spread:
    a) in the direction of hair growth
    c) against the direction of hair growth
    b) as thickly as possible
    d) 3 to 5 times
    _____

23. When waxing, an important rule to remember is to:
    a) pull the fabric strip straight up
    c) double-dip
    b) wear disposable gloves
    d) apply more wax over moles
    _____

24. A temporary hair removal method that produces the same results as hot or cold wax is:
    a) sugaring
    c) shaving
    b) tweezing
    d) electronic tweezing
    _____

Facials

1. All facial cleansing procedures begin with a cleanser and end
   with the application of a/an:
   a) enzyme peel   c) treatment cream
   b) exfoliant   d) tonic lotion   _____

2. For clients who like foaming facial cleansers and a "squeaky
   clean" feeling, you can use a:
   a) face wash   c) cleansing lotion
   b) cleansing cream   d) treatment cream   _____

3. Very dry or mature skin is best cleansed with:
   a) soap and water   c) cleansing cream
   b) face wash   d) cleansing lotion   _____

4. Tonic lotions:
   a) relax the pores   c) are used before cleansing
   b) raise the skin's pH d) remove excess cleanser _____

5. The tonic lotions with the lowest alcohol content are:
   a) tonics   c) astringents
   b) fresheners   d) exfoliants   _____

6. Astringents are used mostly on:
   a) normal skin   c) dry skin
   b) mature skin   d) oily skin   _____

7. Exfoliation is the peeling and shredding of the:
   a) hair follicles   c) adipose layer
   b) horny layer of skin d) dermal layer   _____

8. Mechanical exfoliation products include:
   a) papain peels
   b) alphahydroxy acids
   c) massage creams
   d) granular scrubs _____

9. Microdermabrasion is a method of exfoliation that uses aluminum chloride and other crystals to:
   a) dissolve surface skin cells
   b) abrade the stratum corneum
   c) break down keratin
   d) rub the dead cells off _____

10. Keratolytic enzymes help speed up the breakdown of:
    a) the dermis
    b) collagen
    c) melanin
    d) keratin _____

11. Enzyme peels containing paraffin or oatmeal are also called:
    a) microdermabrasion
    b) vegetable peels
    c) gommage
    d) powdered enzymes _____

12. Enzyme peels that use a powdered form of enzyme:
    a) are not used if acne is present
    b) stay soft during application
    c) dry to a crust
    d) tighten follicle openings _____

13. Alphahydroxy acids are derived mostly from:
    a) gastric acids
    b) quaternary compounds
    c) fruits
    d) beef by-products _____

14. Before a client is exfoliated with alphahydroxy acid, he or she should first use it at home for two weeks in a concentration of:
    a) 5% to 10%
    b) 10% to 20%
    c) 1% to 3%
    d) 20% to 25% _____

15. Treatment creams are used to hydrate and condition the skin:
    a) under makeup
    b) during the night
    c) at the end of a facial
    d) twice a week _____

16. Products ideal for use as a day cream or makeup base are:
    a) nourishing creams
    b) alphahydroxy acids
    c) moisturizers
    d) packs _____

17. Facial masks:
    a) are applied before cleansing
    b) remain soft and creamy on the skin
    c) are all applied over gauze
    d) provide complete closure to the environment   _____

18. One type of facial mask that is melted before application and then hardens on the skin is the:
    a) sulfur mask
    b) clay mask
    c) paraffin mask
    d) modelage mask   _____

19. Clay masks:
    a) harden to a candle-like consistency
    b) grow warmer as they set
    c) contain sulfur
    d) are ready to use   _____

20. If a modelage mask is part of the facial, it is not recommended to:
    a) apply a treatment cream
    b) perform facial massage
    c) cleanse the face first
    d) let the mask cool on the skin   _____

21. Sulfur masks are particularly useful for:
    a) sealing moisture into the skin
    b) treating dry, mature skin
    c) reducing sebum production
    d) stimulating sebum production   _____

22. The purpose of gauze in a facial is to:
    a) prevent a mask from touching the skin
    b) remove packs easily
    c) comply with sanitation laws
    d) hold mask ingredients together   _____

23. Single applications of concentrated extracts to be applied under a night cream or massage cream are contained in:
    a) tubes
    b) droppers
    c) ampules
    d) packs   _____

24. Contraindications for certain facial treatments include the presence of:
    a) metal implants   c) freckles
    b) moles   d) acne   _____

25. Effluerage is a massage movement applied in a:
    a) deep rolling manner with   c) light, slow, rhythmic
       pressure   manner without pressure
    b) heavy tapping manner   d) light pinching manner   _____

26. The direction of a massage movement is always from the muscle's:
    a) attachment toward the   c) origin toward the
       joint   insertion
    b) fixed attachment to its   d) insertion toward its origin   _____
       movable attachment

27. Petrissage is a __ movement.
    a) slapping   c) kneading
    b) rubbing   d) tapping   _____

28. Massage should not be given to clients with high blood pressure or a heart condition because it:
    a) increases circulation   c) requires them to lie flat
    b) may become irritating   d) increases muscular   _____
                                      strength

29. One area the cosmetologist is not licensed to massage is the:
    a) leg below the knee   c) leg above the knee
    b) upper chest   d) below the neck   _____

30. Deep rubbing movements are characteristic of the massage movement called:
    a) tapotement   c) effleurage
    b) friction   d) vibration   _____

31. To master massage techniques, you must have knowledge of anatomy and:
    a) histology   c) chemistry
    b) psychology   d) physiology   _____

32. Firm kneading massage movements usually produce:
    a) soothing sensations   c) muscle contractions
    b) deep stimulation   d) cooling sensations   _____

33. Tapotement is a:
    a) tapping movement   c) squeezing movement
    b) vibratory movement   d) friction movement   _____

34. Wringing is an example of:
    a) kneading   c) fulling
    b) petrissage   d) friction   _____

35. The point on the skin over the muscle where pressure or stimulation will cause contraction of that muscle is called a:
    a) belly   c) motor nerve
    b) motor point   d) sensory nerve   _____

36. Manipulating proper motor points will:
    a) relax the client   c) warm the muscles for
                                   massage
    b) provide the deepest   d) give the skin a glow   _____
       stimulation

37. Normal skin can be maintained by __ massage.
    a) daily   c) weekly
    b) monthly   d) annual   _____

38. Fulling is performed mainly on the:
    a) arms   c) chin
    b) legs   d) neck   _____

39. A form of tapotement used only on the back, shoulders, and arms is:
    a) fulling   c) chucking
    b) hacking   d) tapping   _____

40. The most stimulating massage movement is:
    a) vibration   c) tapotement
    b) kneading   d) friction   _____

41. Every massage should begin and end with:
    a) effleurage   c) vibration
    b) tapotement   d) friction   _____

42. The first product to be used in a plain facial on a female
    client is:
    a) moisturizing lotion   c) eye makeup remover
    b) massage cream   d) an astringent lotion   _____

43. All the modalities used in the salon require two electrodes,
    one negative and one positive, except for:
    a) faradic   c) sinusoidal
    b) high frequency   d) galvanic   _____

44. The applicator for directing the electric current from a
    machine to the client's skin is a/an:
    a) cord   c) electrode
    b) modality   d) insulator   _____

45. A positive electrode:
    a) has a black plug and cord   c) is marked with an "N" or
                                      a minus sign
    b) is called a cathode   d) is marked with a "P" or   _____
                                      plus sign

46. When using the galvanic current, the passive electrode is:
    a) not used on the client's face c) the negative electrode
    b) placed on the left side of   d) used on the area to be   _____
       the body   treated

47. The process of softening and emulsifying grease deposits and
    blackheads in the follicles is called:
    a) ultraviolet therapy   c) desincrustation
    b) iontophoresis   d) anaphoresis   _____

48. Faradic and sinusoidal currents:
    a) force muscles to contract   c) produce chemical changes
    b) are thermal currents   d) have a germicidal effect   _____

49. Electrotherapy that is particularly beneficial for acne-prone skin is applied with a:
    a) faradic current
    b) galvanic current
    c) high-frequency current
    d) sinusoidal current _____

50. A glass electrode that gives off violet sparks operates on a:
    a) galvanic current
    b) high-frequency current
    c) faradic current
    d) sinusoidal current _____

51. When applying and removing a high-frequency current from the skin in a direct surface application:
    a) you must always avoid sparking
    b) the client holds the electrode
    c) hold your finger on the electrode
    d) apply product to the client's face _____

52. The client holds the tube electrode while the cosmetologist massages the client's face in:
    a) indirect high-frequency application
    b) desincrustation
    c) direct high-frequency application
    d) faradic application _____

53. Treatment with light rays is called:
    a) electrotherapy
    b) cataphoresis
    c) heat therapy
    d) light therapy _____

54. The light that produces vitamin D in the skin and can be used to treat rickets, psoriasis, and acne is:
    a) infrared light
    b) ultraviolet light
    c) red light
    d) blue light _____

55. Infrared light:
    a) dilates blood vessels and increases circulation
    b) improves skin tone
    c) increases elimination of waste products
    d) produces germicidal effects _____

56. The two basic types of facials are preservative and:
    a) cleansing
    b) corrective
    c) acne
    d) moisturizing _____

57. Remove facial products from their containers with:
    a) your fingers   c) a spatula
    b) a tissue   d) a spoon   _____

58. When draping for a facial, a towel must be placed:
    a) around the client's feet   c) around the client's neck
    b) on the back of the facial   d) over the client's shoulders   _____
       bed

59. If either exfoliation or eyebrow arching is included in a facial,
    it should be performed:
    a) after makeup is removed   c) before the face is cleansed
    b) after the face is steamed   d) after cleanser is removed   _____
                                      from the face

60. When a facial is given, eye pads should be applied before:
    a) cleansing the face   c) using infrared rays
    b) performing facial   d) applying astringent lotion   _____
       manipulations

61. Following the removal of blackheads during an oily skin
    facial, apply:
    a) cool towels   c) a mud mask
    b) astringent   d) massage cream   _____

62. Once you have started facial manipulations on a client, if it
    becomes necessary to remove your hands:
    a) use feather-like movements   c) use a short, abrupt
                                       movement
    b) apply slight pressure, then   d) do it quickly   _____
       release

63. In a basic facial, the last product to be applied is usually:
    a) tonic lotion or freshener   c) massage cream
    b) moisturizer or sunscreen   d) treatment mask   _____

64. For a client with acne, your role usually is to:
    a) work closely with the   c) provide services you have
       client's physician   tried on others
    b) suggest medical remedies   d) recommend various salon   _____
                                      treatments

65. When skillfully applied, massage benefits the skin by:
   a) warming the skin
   b) increasing circulation
   c) forcing cream into the skin
   d) removing debris   _____

66. When receiving a facial, an important part for the client is the:
   a) lighting
   b) conversation
   c) relaxation
   d) refreshments   _____

67. Clients may be unhappy with a facial service if:
   a) you tell them about future promotions
   b) they do not hear soft music
   c) they see too many products
   d) you run out of products   _____

68. Aromatherapy is defined the therapeutic use of:
   a) candles
   b) dietary oils
   c) essential oils
   d) bath oils   _____

69. When removing blackheads, or comedones, from the skin:
   a) press from under the follicle
   b) use your fingernails to squeeze
   c) use bare hands for better control
   d) use your thumbs to squeeze   _____

70. When applying faradic or sinusoidal currents, place the cathode on the:
   a) origin of the muscle
   b) belly of the muscle
   c) fixed attachment of the muscle
   d) insertion of the muscle   _____

Facial Makeup

1. The cosmetic used as a base or as a protective film is:
   a) foundation
   b) cheek color
   c) powder
   d) concealer   _____

2. Water-based cream-to-powder foundation is particularly effective for:
   a) dry skin
   b) normal skin
   c) oily skin
   d) all skin types   _____

3. Pot concealer:
   a) may double as foundation
   b) provides the most coverage
   c) provides sheer to medium coverage
   d) is fluid in consistency   _____

4. The cosmetic that adds a matte or dull finish to the face is:
   a) powder
   b) cheek color
   c) moisturizer
   d) concealer   _____

5. Translucent face powder is:
   a) the same color as foundation
   b) darker than foundation
   c) lighter than foundation
   d) colorless   _____

6. The cosmetic also known as blush, blusher, or rouge is:
   a) cheek color
   b) foundation
   c) concealer
   d) face powder   _____

7. Lip color should be applied with a lip brush beginning:
   a) at the peak of the upper lip
   b) at the corner of the lower lip
   c) in the middle of the lower lip
   d) at the outer corner of the upper lip _____

8. Lip liner helps to keep lip color from:
   a) fading
   b) looking too dark
   c) feathering
   d) drying out _____

9. When applying eye shadow, you should as a rule avoid:
   a) matching eye shadow to eye color
   b) coordinating eye shadow with clothing
   c) use light and dark eye shadow together
   d) using eye shadow darker than iris color _____

10. An eye shadow that is darker and deeper than the client's skin tone is called a:
   a) highlight color
   b) neutral color
   c) contour color
   d) base color _____

11. Eyeliner is used to make the:
   a) lashes look longer
   b) eyes appear larger
   c) lash color match the brow color
   d) natural color of the iris appear darker _____

12. To apply a line close to the lash line with a softer effect, you may use:
   a) eyebrow pencil
   b) dark foundation
   c) eye shadow
   d) mascara _____

13. When applying eyebrow color, avoid:
   a) applying it after tweezing or waxing
   b) harsh contrasts between hair and eyebrow color
   c) filling in sparse areas
   d) lightening the eyebrows _____

14. Mascara is not available in:
   a) pencil form
   b) cake form
   c) liquid form
   d) cream form _____

15. An angle brush may be used to apply:
    a) blusher
    b) lip color
    c) eyebrow shadow
    d) concealer _____

16. Blues, greens, and violets are:
    a) cool colors
    b) secondary colors
    c) warm colors
    d) complementary colors _____

17. The three main factors to consider when choosing makeup colors for a client are skin color, eye color, and:
    a) clothing color
    b) hair color
    c) nail color
    d) eyebrow color _____

18. Complementary colors for blue eyes include:
    a) pinks and plums
    b) grays and silvers
    c) peach and copper
    d) greens and blues _____

19. When choosing makeup colors for a client, avoid:
    a) mixing warm and cool colors
    b) using neutral colors
    c) using all cool colors
    d) using all warm colors _____

20. Before applying foundation makeup:
    a) the skin should be moistened
    b) lip color is selected
    c) the skin should be cleansed
    d) face powder is applied _____

21. The color of foundation is tested by blending on a client's:
    a) forehead
    b) jawline
    c) eyelid
    d) wrist _____

22. The last cosmetic to be applied is usually:
    a) cheek color
    b) face powder
    c) mascara
    d) lip color _____

23. In corrective makeup, a lighter shade of foundation:
    a) minimizes a facial area
    b) emphasizes a facial area
    c) conceals blemishes
    d) widens or lengthens an area _____

24. The primary objective of corrective makeup is to create the optical illusion of a/an:
    a) oval face
    b) heart-shaped face
    c) round face
    d) diamond-shaped face _____

25. A client with an inverted triangle (heart-shaped) face can be identified by:
    a) a high forehead
    b) a jawline wider than the forehead
    c) a narrow forehead
    d) a narrow jawline and a wide forehead _____

26. Corrective makeup for a large or protruding nose includes:
    a) darker foundation on the nose
    b) lighter foundation on the nose
    c) darker foundation on cheeks beside the nose
    d) cheek color placed close to the nose _____

27. To minimize wide-set eyes and make them appear closer, it is best to:
    a) make the eyebrow line straight
    b) shorten outside eyebrow line on both sides
    c) extend eyebrow lines to inside corners of eyes
    d) arch the ends of the eyebrows _____

28. Ruddy skin can be corrected with a foundation that is:
    a) yellow
    b) reddish
    c) peach
    d) pink _____

29. Band lashes are:
    a) made only of human or animal hair
    b) applied before eyeliner
    c) attached to the lids one at a time
    d) attached to a strip _____

30. Eye tabbing involves:
    a) tinting eyelashes
    b) applying individual lashes
    c) removing artificial lashes
    d) applying strip eyelashes _____

Nail Structure and Growth

1. The nails are an appendage of the:
   a) hair
   b) muscles
   c) skin
   d) skeleton
   _____

2. A healthy nail appears:
   a) slightly pink
   b) yellowish
   c) slightly purple
   d) light blue
   _____

3. The technical name for the nail is:
   a) onychauxis
   b) onyx
   c) onychosis
   d) onychia
   _____

4. The nail is composed mainly of:
   a) keratin
   b) collagen
   c) melanin
   d) sebum
   _____

5. The nail has between __ water content.
   a) 50% and 75%
   b) 5% and 10%
   c) 30% and 50%
   d) 10% and 30%
   _____

6. The portion of the skin on which the nail plate rests is the:
   a) lunula
   b) nail plate
   c) nail bed
   d) matrix bed
   _____

7. The nail is formed in the:
   a) mantle
   b) matrix bed (nail root)
   c) nail bed
   d) hyponychium
   _____

8. The visible portion of the matrix bed (nail root) is called the:
   - a) mantle
   - b) bed epithelium
   - c) lunula
   - d) nail groove
   _____

9. The most visible and functional part of the nail unit is the:
   - a) hyponychium
   - b) nail plate
   - c) matrix bed
   - d) free edge
   _____

10. The area around the base of the fingernails and toenails is sealed against foreign material and microorganisms by the:
    - a) cuticle
    - b) nail groove
    - c) nail fold
    - d) ligament
    _____

11. The cuticle overlapping the lunula is the:
    - a) nail fold
    - b) mantle
    - c) eponychium
    - d) hyponychium
    _____

12. The portion of the skin under the free edge is called the:
    - a) mantle
    - b) eponychium
    - c) cuticle
    - d) hyponychium
    _____

13. The part of the nail that extends over the fingertip is the:
    - a) cuticle
    - b) hyponychium
    - c) free edge
    - d) lunula
    _____

14. The nail bed and matrix bed are attached to the underlying bone by:
    - a) the bed epithelium
    - b) nail grooves
    - c) muscles
    - d) ligaments
    _____

15. The deep fold of skin in which the matrix bed is embedded is the:
    - a) nail groove
    - b) mantle
    - c) hyponichium
    - d) nail fold
    _____

16. In an adult, nails grow at an average rate of:
    - a) 1/8" per month
    - b) 1/8" per week
    - c) 1/4" per week
    - d) 1/2" per month
    _____

17. One nail condition that may receive a manicure is:
    a) onychia   c) paronychia
    b) onychophagy   d) onychosis   _____

18. Abnormal brittleness or splitting of the nails may be caused by:
    a) overuse of cuticle oil   c) nail polish
    b) hangnails   d) careless filing   _____

19. White spots on the nails are known as:
    a) hangnails   c) onychauxis
    b) leukonychia   d) onychatrophia   _____

20. When the cuticle splits around the nail, it is known as:
    a) pterygium   c) onychophagy
    b) hangnails   d) onychorrhexis   _____

21. Blue nails are often a sign of:
    a) poor blood circulation   c) a lung disorder
    b) a stomach ailment   d) a finger infection   _____

22. Wavy ridges on the nails are caused by:
    a) careless filing of the nails   c) dryness of the cuticle
    b) uneven growth of the nails   d) biting the nails   _____

23. When manicuring a client with corrugations, you can buff the nails carefully and use a:
    a) antiseptic cream   c) ridge filler
    b) harsh abrasive   d) coat of primer   _____

24. Hangnails can be caused by:
    a) improper diet   c) local infection
    b) cutting off too much cuticle   d) injury to the base of the   _____
                                      nail

25. Eggshell nails are thinner and __ than normal.
    a) less fragile   c) more flexible
    b) more rigid   d) darker   _____

26. Melanonychia may be seen under or within the nail plate as a:
    a) purplish spot
    c) white spot
    b) yellow-green spot
    d) black band   _____

27. The atrophy or wasting away of the nail is called:
    a) onychoptosis
    c) melanonychia
    b) onychatrophia
    d) felon   _____

28. An abnormal overgrowth of the nail is known as:
    a) atrophy
    c) onychorrhexis
    b) onychophagy
    d) hypertrophy   _____

29. "Folded nail," a disorder characterized by one or both edges of the nail plate folded at 90 degrees or more into the soft tissues of the nail margins, is also called:
    a) onychauxis
    c) pterygium
    b) plicatured nail
    d) trumpet nail   _____

30. Abnormally brittle nails with striations are a disorder called:
    a) onychorrhexis
    c) agnails
    b) furrows
    d) onychophagy   _____

31. A client with pterygium will have one or more nails with:
    a) wavy ridges
    c) whitish discoloration
    b) abnormal brittleness
    d) forward growth of the   _____
       eponychium

32. An increased crosswise curvature throughout the nail plate is a symptom of:
    a) tile-shaped nails
    c) plicatured nails
    b) eggshell nails
    d) trumpet nails   _____

33. Discolorations between the nail plate and artificial enhancements, which used to be called "molds," are actually caused by:
    a) fungi
    c) bacteria
    b) viruses
    d) injury   _____

34. Do not perform nail services for clients who have:
    a) leukonychia
    b) fungus on their nails
    c) abnormally brittle nails
    d) forward growth of the
       eponychium   _____

35. The general term for vegetable parasites is:
    a) fungi
    b) flagella
    c) tinea
    d) onychosis   _____

36. Pseudomonas aeruginosa is a type of:
    a) virus
    b) overgrowth
    c) bacteria
    d) nail shedding   _____

37. The technical term indicating any nail disease or deformity is:
    a) onychosis
    b) onyx
    c) onychophagy
    d) onychauxis   _____

38. People who work with their hands in water or who must
    wash their hands continually are prone to:
    a) onychoptosis
    b) pyogenic granuloma
    c) onychogryposis
    d) paronychia   _____

39. Onychia is an inflammation with pus formation affecting the:
    a) matrix bed
    b) nail body
    c) free edge
    d) cuticles   _____

40. The technical term for ingrown nails is:
    a) onychia
    b) felon
    c) onychocryptosis
    d) tinea   _____

41. Onychogryposis is most commonly seen on the:
    a) middle finger
    b) thumb
    c) little toe
    d) great toe   _____

42. The loosening of the nail without shedding, usually from the
    free edge to the lunula, is called:
    a) onychomadesis
    b) onychogryposis
    c) onycholysis
    d) onychia   _____

43. Onychomadesis, onychoptosis, and onychia all have this symptom in common:
    a) shedding of the nail
    b) blisters on the skin
    c) overgrowth of the nail
    d) inflammation of the nail   _____

44. The common name for tinea is:
    a) felon
    b) ringworm
    c) ingrown nails
    d) hangnail   _____

45. A severe inflammation of the nail in which a lump of red tissue grows from the nail bed to the nail plate is known as:
    a) onychophagy
    b) paronychia
    c) pyogenic granuloma
    d) onychauxis   _____

46. The medical term for athlete's foot is:
    a) tinea unguium
    b) tinea favosa
    c) tinea capitis
    d) tinea pedis   _____

47. Tinea unguium is commonly called:
    a) ringworm of the scalp
    b) ringworm of the nails
    c) honeycomb ringworm
    d) athlete's foot   _____

48. One common form of tinea unguium is characterized by:
    a) whitish patches on the nail surface
    b) a lump of red tissue
    c) blisters under the nail
    d) shedding nails   _____

49. An infected finger should be treated by a/an:
    a) instructor
    b) nail technician
    c) cosmetologist
    d) physician   _____

50. The only service you may be allowed to perform for a client with nail fungus is to:
    a) refill the new growth
    b) apply polish
    c) remove any artificial nails
    d) buff to a shine   _____

Manicuring and Pedicuring

1. The permanent tools you use to perform nail services are collectively called:
   a) implements
   b) equipment
   c) materials
   d) nail cosmetics
   _____

2. Cotton balls and liquid soap used in a manicure service are classified as:
   a) equipment
   b) nail cosmetics
   c) materials
   d) implements
   _____

3. The adjustable lamp for a manicure table should have a __ bulb.
   a) 25-watt
   b) 40-watt
   c) 75-watt
   d) 60-watt
   _____

4. Reusable implements include:
   a) cuticle pushers
   b) emery boards
   c) orangewood sticks
   d) chamois covers
   _____

5. Before used implements are placed in disinfectant, they must be:
   a) rinsed in alcohol
   b) cleaned with a paper towel
   c) cleaned in an autoclave
   d) washed with soap and water
   _____

6. Emery boards are used to:
   a) shape the free edge
   b) remove dirt from under the nail
   c) thin the free edge
   d) push back the cuticle
   _____

7. If blood is drawn during a procedure, the implement should be:
   - a) rinsed with water
   - b) discarded
   - c) cleaned and disinfected
   - d) wiped off with cotton

   _____

8. Brittle nails and dry cuticles are treated with a/an:
   - a) cuticle pusher
   - b) extended soaking time
   - c) hand massage
   - d) oil manicure

   _____

9. A nail hardener is applied:
   - a) after the base coat
   - b) after the nail polish
   - c) after the top coat
   - d) before the base coat

   _____

10. A manicure that is not given in the manicuring area, and often is given while the client is receiving another service, is called a:
    - a) plain manicure
    - b) hot oil manicure
    - c) booth manicure
    - d) mobile manicure

    _____

11. Fresh disinfectant solution for implements should be prepared:
    - a) every 2 days
    - b) weekly
    - c) 3 times a day
    - d) daily

    _____

12. When shaping the fingernail, file the nail from:
    - a) corner to center
    - b) left to right
    - c) center to corner
    - d) corner to corner

    _____

13. Polish should be removed from the nail with:
    - a) a firm movement from tip to base
    - b) a twisting motion
    - c) a circular motion
    - d) a firm movement from base to tip

    _____

14. All traces of oil must be removed after an oil manicure before:
    - a) massage
    - b) filing
    - c) applying the base coat
    - d) applying the top coat

    _____

15. A hand massage may be given before:
    - a) soaking fingers
    - b) filing
    - c) pushing cuticles
    - d) polish

    _____

16. Once polish has been applied, wipe away excess with:
    a) your thumbnail
    b) a cuticle pusher
    c) a cotton-tipped orangewood stick
    d) a cotton pledget _____

17. Apply nail polish:
    a) before the base coat
    b) over the sealer
    c) over the top coat
    d) over the base coat _____

18. The ideal nail shape is:
    a) pointed
    b) oval
    c) round
    d) square _____

19. Stains on fingernails may be removed with nail bleach or:
    a) peroxide
    b) an oil manicure
    c) dry nail polish
    d) acetone _____

20. An optional step in a manicure is to apply nail bleach:
    a) on top of the free edge
    b) around the cuticle
    c) under the free edge
    d) over the nail bed _____

21. A top coat or sealer makes the nail polish:
    a) adhere to the nail surface
    b) dry quickly
    c) appear thicker
    d) more resistant to chipping _____

22. If a client has athlete's foot, recommend:
    a) a medicated shoe insert
    b) a pedicure
    c) a physician's examination
    d) changing socks more frequently _____

23. If offering a leg massage with a pedicure, do not massage:
    a) below the knee
    b) the side of the shinbone
    c) above the ankle
    d) the shinbone _____

24. A physician who treats diseases of the feet is known as a/an:
    a) ophthalmologist
    b) podiatrist
    c) dermatologist
    d) orthopedic physician _____

25. If a client is accidentally cut during a manicure, apply:
    a) alcohol
    b) styptic pencil
    c) powdered alum
    d) disinfectant _____

26. To mix nail polish:
    - a) stir the polish with the brush
    - b) strike the bottle against your palm
    - c) shake the bottle
    - d) roll the bottle between your palms _____

27. In a French manicure, the free edge of the nail is polished, tipped, or sculpted in a/an:
    - a) translucent color
    - b) opaque color
    - c) clear polish
    - d) dark color _____

28. A French manicure differs from an American manicure in that the French manicure uses __ on the free edge.
    - a) a translucent pink
    - b) a pale, opaque pink
    - c) a more dramatic white
    - d) a more subtle white _____

29. In a man's manicure, the nails are often finished with:
    - a) base coat
    - b) flowery hand cream
    - c) cuticle oil
    - d) dry polish _____

30. The nail hardener that uses keratin fibers to strengthen the nail is:
    - a) formaldehyde hardener
    - b) keratin hardener
    - c) protein hardener
    - d) nylon fiber hardener _____

31. One of the functions of base coat is to prevent nail polish from:
    - a) adhering to the nail plate
    - b) forming a high gloss
    - c) adhering to the nail bed
    - d) staining the nail plate _____

32. The product that contains moisturizing ingredients and is used independently of a manicure is:
    - a) nail conditioner
    - b) hand lotion
    - c) cuticle oil
    - d) cuticle cream _____

33. Nail dryer protects the nail polish against:
    - a) staining the nail plate
    - b) too high a gloss
    - c) stickiness and dulling
    - d) adhering to the nail surface _____

34. The two parts of a consultation for a manicure service are the analysis and:
a) filling out the client record
b) a sales pitch
c) the service itself
d) the recommendations _____

35. The squoval nail shape is:
a) round with the corners squared
b) square with the ends rounded
c) tapered with the tip squared
d) oval with the ends squared _____

36. A consultation for a manicure service takes place after:
a) you clean up your work area
b) the hand massage
c) you have removed old polish
d) the client washes her hands _____

37. Be sure to check with your instructor or your regulatory agency about:
a) loosening the cuticle
b) reusing emery boards
c) nipping cuticles or hangnails
d) using nail clippers _____

38. Calluses at the fingertips can be treated with creams and lotions or by:
a) careful trimming with nail scissors
b) filing them down
c) dissolving with chemicals
d) rubbing with pumice powder _____

39. An optional implement used to remove dry, flaky skin and smooth calluses on the foot is the:
a) foot file
b) nail rasp
c) diamond nail file
d) curette _____

40. Calluses on the feet:
a) should be left alone
b) require medical treatment
c) should be removed
d) protect the underlying skin _____

Advanced Nail Techniques

1. After washing implements with soap and warm water:
   - a) store them in a sealed container
   - b) rinse away all soap
   - c) dry them thoroughly
   - d) place them in disinfectant _____

2. During the preservice procedure, working surfaces should be sprayed with a/an:
   - a) antiseptic
   - b) household bleach
   - c) EPA-registered disinfectant
   - d) alcohol solution _____

3. Nail tips:
   - a) are temporary with or without overlay
   - b) cover no more than half the nail plate
   - c) cover the entire nail plate
   - d) can be made of silk or linen _____

4. A substance that should never be used on plastic artificial nails is:
   - a) hand lotion
   - b) cuticle oil
   - c) acetone polish remover
   - d) nail polish dryer _____

5. The "stop, rock, and hold" procedure is used to apply:
   - a) fiberglass wraps
   - b) acrylic nails over forms
   - c) light-cured gels
   - d) nail tips _____

6. Removing softened nail tips is done by:
   - a) sliding them off
   - b) pulling them off
   - c) rubbing them off
   - d) dissolving them completely _____

7. To protect a client's damaged or fragile nails, you may recommend:
   a) an oil manicure
   b) cuticle pushing
   c) nail filing
   d) nail wrapping   _____

8. Nail wraps using silk:
   a) are rarely used
   b) are very thick
   c) give a smooth, even appearance
   d) have a loose weave   _____

9. The nail wraps that must be reapplied when polish is removed are:
   a) fiberglass wraps
   b) silk wraps
   c) linen wraps
   d) paper wraps   _____

10. To remove any natural oil and dehydrate the nail for better adhesion of tips and nail wraps, use a/an:
    a) nail adhesive
    b) adhesive dryer
    c) nail antiseptic
    d) primer   _____

11. After placing nail wrap material on the nail, apply adhesive to the:
    a) top of the nail only
    b) entire nail
    c) cuticles
    d) free edge only   _____

12. Fabric wraps require glue and fabric fills after:
    a) 2 months
    b) 2 weeks
    c) 4 weeks
    d) 6 weeks   _____

13. A nail tip is very weak if it is worn with no:
    a) overlay
    b) adhesive
    c) polish
    d) buffing   _____

14. The point at which the nail plate meets the nail tip before the tip is glued to the nail is known as the:
    a) well
    b) tip stop
    c) position stop
    d) contact point   _____

15. Liquid nail wrap contains:
    a) liquid acrylic
    b) tiny fibers
    c) extra adhesive
    d) protein   _____

16. Artificial nails created by combining a liquid acrylic product with a powdered product are:
    a) gel nails   c) dipped nails
    b) fiberglass nails   d) acrylic nails   _____

17. A substance made up of many small molecules that are not attached to one another is known as a:
    a) monomer   c) polymer
    b) catalyst   d) primer   _____

18. The substance that improves the adhesion between an acrylic nail and the natural nail is the:
    a) nail antiseptic   c) catalyst
    b) overlay   d) primer   _____

19. When applying acrylic, the first ball should be placed:
    a) at one side of the nail   c) at the base of the nail
    b) at the free edge   d) in the middle of the nail _____

20. The third ball in an acrylic nail application should be:
    a) spread thickly near the   c) extremely wet
       cuticle
    b) placed just below the first d) more powder than liquid _____
       ball

21. Brushes used with acrylic are cleaned by dipping into:
    a) soapy water   c) alcohol
    b) a weak quat   d) polish remover   _____

22. To help prevent contamination in an acrylic nail service, do not touch the nail:
    a) after dust and filings are   c) after primer is applied
       removed
    b) after the base coat has   d) with bare hands   _____
       dried

23. The trapping of dirt and __ between sculptured nails and the natural nail may lead to bacterial infection.
    a) natural nail oils   c) primer
    b) nail polish   d) moisture   _____

24. Gel nails are artificial nails that are applied by:
    a) dabbing and pressing to the
       nail plate
    b) the stop, rock, and hold
       method
    c) brushing onto the nail
       plate
    d) gluing to the nail plate   _____

25. Light-cured gels harden when they are exposed to:
    a) infrared light
    b) ultraviolet or halogen
    c) sunlight
    d) incandescent light   _____

The Salon Business

1. In a booth rental (also called chair rental) arrangement, the
   stylist is responsible for all the following except:
   a) clientele   c) supplies
   b) accounting   d) mortgage payments   _____

2. Booth rental (or chair rental) is different from salon
   ownership in that with booth rental:
   a) the initial investment is   c) you do not have to keep
       larger   records
   b) you carry your own   d) overhead is slightly higher   _____
       insurance

3. When selecting the location for a salon, you should consider:
   a) the direct competition   c) the number of staff to
                                    hire
   b) the hair services you will   d) your personnel policies   _____
       offer

4. Information about the size, average income, and buying
   habits of the population is called:
   a) a charter   c) a business plan
   b) a census   d) demographics   _____

5. Before you seek financing to open a salon, you must first
   develop a:
   a) color scheme   c) charter
   b) business plan   d) brochure   _____

6. Building renovations and business codes are regulated by:
   a) local regulations
   b) federal laws
   c) state or province laws
   d) the department of licensing

   _____

7. Social Security is covered under:
   a) local laws
   b) state or province laws
   c) federal laws
   d) county laws

   _____

8. Salon owners purchase insurance policies to protect themselves against:
   a) loss of employees
   b) malpractice lawsuits
   c) loss of clients
   d) increases in rent

   _____

9. A salon that is owned by stockholders and has a state charter is a/an:
   a) partnership
   b) individual ownership
   c) corporation
   d) joint ownership

   _____

10. The type of ownership that subjects the owner to the most limited personal loss is the:
    a) individual ownership
    b) corporation
    c) partnership
    d) co-ownership

    _____

11. If two people own a salon together, that type of ownership is a/an:
    a) partnership
    b) individual ownership
    c) chain salon
    d) corporation

    _____

12. If you lease a space for your salon, the lease should specify who is responsible for:
    a) employee benefits
    b) repairs
    c) income taxes
    d) advertising

    _____

13. Before you open a business, you need to determine how much capital you will need to run it for at least the first:
    a) two years
    b) six months
    c) five years
    d) one year

    _____

14. Quality control means that every time clients come to the salon they can expect:
    a) the same stylist   c) the same products used
    b) consistently high standards d) a different haircut   _____

15. Receipts from services and retail sales are classified as:
    a) income   c) expenses
    b) client records   d) outgo   _____

16. For the average salon, the net profit is about __ of the total gross income.
    a) 85 percent   c) 50 percent
    b) 25 percent   d) 15 percent   _____

17. Information about which products are selling well and which ones are not can be seen in the salon's:
    a) inventory records   c) consumption records
    b) petty cash book   d) service records   _____

18. Major purchases of supplies should be made:
    a) when they are needed   c) after tax time
    b) when suppliers offer special d) before filing income taxes _____
       prices

19. For satisfactory client service, it is essential that the salon have good plumbing and:
    a) public transportation   c) parking facilities
    b) office space   d) lighting   _____

20. Guidelines that require that the ingredients of cosmetic preparations be displayed prominently for clients are put out by:
    a) state or province boards c) OSHA
    b) the Department of   d) the EPA   _____
       Education

21. The best form of advertising is:
    a) a neon sign   c) a newspaper ad
    b) satisfied clients   d) window displays   _____

22. Closer contact is made with potential clients by using:
    a) direct mail advertising   c) radio advertising
    b) newspaper advertising   d) yellow pages advertising _____

23. The largest expense item in operating a salon is:
    a) supplies   c) salaries
    b) rent   d) advertising _____

24. The "quarterback" of the salon is the:
    a) stylist   c) shampoo person
    b) receptionist   d) manager _____

25. An accurate reflection of what is taking place in the salon at
    a given time can be seen in:
    a) an income tax return   c) yearly records
    b) its business plan   d) the appointment book _____

26. Salon and individual licenses are covered by:
    a) state or province laws   c) local laws
    b) federal laws   d) county laws _____

27. When booking appointments by telephone in the salon, you
    should:
    a) give most clients to an   c) give most clients to a new
       established stylist   stylist
    b) be familiar with all services d) use a pencil in case of _____
       and products   cancellations

28. When listening to a client's complaint, it is important to
    avoid:
    a) interrupting   c) being sympathetic
    b) apologizing   d) promising free service _____

29. Client records should be kept:
    a) in the dispensary   c) at your station
    b) in the office   d) at a central location _____

30. The approximate percentage of a salon's budget spent on
    salaries is:
    a) 25   c) 50
    b) 75   d) 35 _____

31. Products that are sold to clients are:
    a) consumption supplies   c) wholesale supplies
    b) stock supplies   d) retail supplies   _____

32. Local, state or province, and federal tax laws require a
    business to maintain:
    a) an advertising budget   c) a parking area
    b) proper business records   d) a dress code for   _____
                                     employees

33. In order to maintain an accurate and efficient control of
    supplies, it is necessary to have an organized:
    a) service record   c) inventory system
    b) security system   d) purchase system   _____

34. Salon supplies that are used in the daily business operation
    are called:
    a) retail supplies   c) inventory
    b) wholesale supplies   d) consumption supplies   _____

35. Payroll books and canceled checks should be retained for:
    a) seven months   c) 10 years
    b) seven years   d) one year   _____

36. In the allotment of funds, the top priority should always be
    paying the:
    a) suppliers   c) employees
    b) insurance   d) rent   _____

37. Guidelines for becoming an effective manager include:
    a) sharing information   c) delaying feedback
    b) letting employees learn on d) doubting employees'   _____
       their own   intentions

38. Advertising should be concentrated around:
    a) your personal schedule   c) newspaper schedules
    b) the holidays   d) slow periods   _____

39. In general, your advertising budget should not be greater
    than __ of your total gross income.
    a) 3 percent   c) 10 percent
    b) 1 percent   d) 5 percent   _____

40. An important point to keep in mind when retailing is to recommend to clients:

a) what works best for you

b) the more expensive products

c) everything in a product line

d) what is in their best interest _____

Seeking Employment

1. Motivation, energy, and persistence set apart:
   a) followers
   b) unambitious people
   c) successful people
   d) the overambitious   _____

2. Before you can obtain a job in the cosmetology field, you must:
   a) buy a new wardrobe
   b) pass a licensing exam
   c) work for no pay
   d) plan your whole career   _____

3. A good test-taker prepares by practicing good study habits, including:
   a) taking effective notes
   b) studying when you can fit it in
   c) cramming the night before
   d) skimming the material   _____

4. When taking a test, a helpful strategy is to:
   a) work a question until complete
   b) cram the night before
   c) skim the entire test before beginning
   d) work very fast   _____

5. Deductive reasoning is the process of:
   a) reaching logical conclusions
   b) guessing the answer
   c) relying on intuition
   d) memorizing the right answers   _____

6. The single most important factor in preparing successfully for a test is to:
   a) review past quizzes
   b) make yourself mentally ready
   c) know the material thoroughly
   d) take notes _____

7. When taking a true/false exam, remember:
   a) absolutes are usually true
   b) to watch for qualifying words
   c) to outline your answer first
   d) to choose the short statement _____

8. When you take a multiple-choice test:
   a) answer only if you're positive
   b) stop reading at the right answer
   c) read the questions and choices carefully
   d) avoid "all of the above" _____

9. In order to be prepared for the practical portion of the licensing exam:
   a) clean your implements at the exam site
   b) watch what the other test takers are doing
   c) follow the instructions loosely
   d) do a practice exam _____

10. Willingness to work hard is a key ingredient to success, and later in the workplace:
   a) other people will slack off
   b) your energy will be rewarded
   c) you'll burn out
   d) people will take advantage of you _____

11. Personal characteristics that will help you get the position you want include all the following except:
   a) motivation
   b) integrity
   c) enthusiasm
   d) self-importance _____

12. A small independent salon is often owned and managed by a:
   a) hairstylist
   b) franchise owner
   c) chain
   d) syndicate of owners _____

13. A series of ten or less salons owned by one or two individuals
    is considered a/an:
    a) small independent salon   c) independent salon chain
    b) franchise salon   d) basic value-priced
                                      operation   _____

14. A written summary of your education and work experience is
    called a:
    a) summary   c) abstract
    b) resume   d) data sheet   _____

15. An important guideline when creating a resume is to:
    a) keep it simple and brief   c) make it very detailed
    b) list all education and work d) use bright-colored paper _____
       experience

16. The best way to write accomplishment statements in your
    resume that focus on your achievements is to:
    a) detail prior duties   c) list hobbies and
                                      memberships
    b) use numbers and   d) state your salary history _____
       percentages

17. The do's of resume writing include all the following except:
    a) emphasize transferable   c) make it easy to read
       skills
    b) know your audience   d) enclose a photo   _____

18. A collection of photos and documents reflecting your skills,
    accomplishments, and abilities is called a:
    a) portfolio   c) attachè case
    b) diploma   d) resume   _____

19. When searching for your first job, it's wise to:
    a) go for the perfect job   c) take any job you can get
    b) wait until you have a   d) begin before graduation   _____
       diploma

20. A salon visit, as part of networking, allows you to:
    a) critique the operations   c) get a job offer
    b) observe the operations   d) get a free service   _____

21. Once you're ready for a job interview, the first step in contacting the salons you're interested in is to:
    a) pay a surprise visit
    b) make a phone call
    c) send a resume and cover letter
    d) wait to hear from them _____

22. An important part of going to an interview is to:
    a) wear dressy clothes
    b) take tranquilizers
    c) carry handbag and briefcase
    d) bring supporting materials _____

23. An important behavior to remember at the job interview is to:
    a) be punctual
    b) remain serious
    c) project an informal attitude
    d) smoke in the smoking area _____

24. During a job interview there are some types of questions that are illegal, such as:
    a) education background
    b) date of birth
    c) drug use
    d) employment history _____

25. "Down time" between appointments in a salon can be put to productive use by:
    a) reading industry journals
    b) gossiping with the working stylists
    c) relaxing at your station
    d) criticizing coworkers _____

On the Job

1. In order to be successful, it is important to accept a position at a salon that:
   a) expects the minimum from you
   b) pays the highest wage
   c) makes the first offer
   d) matches your personal style _____

2. If you have a commitment during certain hours or days of the week that might interfere with your work schedule, the best approach at the interview is to:
   a) discuss it frankly
   b) hope it doesn't interfere
   c) expect your coworkers to cover
   d) deal with it later _____

3. One entry-level job for a new graduate is:
   a) receptionist
   b) manager
   c) assistant
   d) color services specialist _____

4. In the service-oriented cosmetology field, a helpful guideline is:
   a) leave if problems arise
   b) be therapist and advisor
   c) put yourself first
   d) put others first _____

5. Working in a salon requires that you practice people skills, including all of the following except:
   a) being a problem solver
   b) being best friends with everyone
   c) being loyal
   d) remaining positive _____

6. When you take a job, you will be expected to perform certain duties and responsibilities, which are described in a:
   a) job description
   b) training manual
   c) legal contract
   d) conversation with your manager _____

7. In a beginning position the best way to be compensated is by:
   a) under the table
   b) commission
   c) tips only
   d) salary _____

8. One form of compensation is commission, which represents:
   a) tips
   b) a percentage of sales
   c) an hourly wage
   d) salary plus percentage _____

9. Tips are income in addition to your regular compensation and:
   a) are taxable at 50%
   b) are not taxable
   c) must be reported as income
   d) are declared but not taxed _____

10. Evaluations, which are commonly scheduled after 90 days for new employees, are meant to provide:
    a) feedback on performance
    b) negative criticism
    c) promotions
    d) raises _____

11. Identifying a role model who is having the kind of success you wish to have:
    a) takes away your individuality
    b) is unfair competition
    c) is imitation
    d) helps improve your performance _____

12. The process of learning how to deal with your money in a constructive way is known as:
    a) thriftiness
    b) managing debt
    c) financial planning
    d) getting credit _____

13. When borrowing money, it is irresponsible and immature to:
    a) default
    b) invest the money
    c) use it for luxuries
    d) pay it back _____

14. Budgeting is a way to:
    - a) save money
    - b) invest money
    - c) estimate income and expenses
    - d) restrict your spending _____

15. Keeping track of where your money goes is a step toward:
    - a) being stingy
    - b) limiting spending
    - c) never having surprises
    - d) always having enough _____

16. When it's not realistic to ask for a raise or higher commission rate, you can increase your income by:
    - a) taking cash from the register
    - b) playing the lottery
    - c) spending less money
    - d) taking others' clients _____

17. Ticket upgrading or upselling is the practice of:
    - a) charging for services not requested
    - b) overcharging
    - c) taking advantage of the client
    - d) recommending additional services _____

18. The practice of retailing consists of:
    - a) recommending additional services
    - b) misrepresenting products
    - c) recommending and selling products
    - d) selling yourself _____

19. To be successful in sales requires ambition, determination, and:
    - a) boldness
    - b) insincerity
    - c) aggression
    - d) a good personality _____

20. The principles of successful sales include all of the following except:
    - a) know your products
    - b) demonstrate use if possible
    - c) always use a soft sell approach
    - d) never misrepresent your product _____

21. When retailing products to your clients, practice all the following except:
   a) asking what products they use
   b) telling them what they need
   c) describing a product's benefits
   d) mentioning any sales _____

22. To build a successful career in cosmetology, it is vital to build a client base, which consists of:
   a) one-time customers
   b) walk-in customers
   c) first-time customers
   d) steady customers _____

23. An important point to keep in mind when building a client base is:
   a) always being positive
   b) rushing clients through their service
   c) developing intimate personal relationships
   d) recommending all sale products _____

24. An inexpensive, easy marketing technique that can help build your client base is:
   a) word of mouth
   b) business card referrals
   c) advertising balloons
   d) newspaper inserts _____

25. The best time to get your client back for the next appointment is:
   a) two weeks before she is due back
   b) a week before she is due back
   c) while she is still in your chair
   d) when she needs new services _____

ANSWER KEY

HISTORY OF COSMETOLOGY

1. A	6. B	11. D	16. D	21. D
2. A	7. A	12. C	17. B	22. B
3. D	8. B	13. B	18. A	23. B
4. D	9. B	14. B	19. D	24. B
5. A	10. A	15. B	20. A	25. A

LIFE SKILLS

1. A	6. A	11. A	16. A	21. B
2. D	7. B	12. D	17. D	22. C
3. B	8. C	13. B	18. B	23. C
4. C	9. A	14. B	19. B	24. C
5. A	10. D	15. C	20. D	25. A

YOUR PROFESSIONAL IMAGE

1. C	6. C	11. D	16. D	21. B
2. D	7. A	12. D	17. B	22. B
3. D	8. B	13. A	18. C	23. B
4. B	9. B	14. A	19. A	24. B
5. C	10. A	15. A	20. A	25. B

COMMUNICATING FOR SUCCESS

1. C	6. D	11. C	16. D	21. A
2. B	7. C	12. B	17. C	22. D
3. A	8. C	13. D	18. A	23. C
4. B	9. C	14. A	19. A	24. B
5. C	10. B	15. D	20. A	25. A

INFECTION CONTROL: PRINCIPLES AND PRACTICE

1. C	14. A	27. C	40. D	53. A
2. B	15. B	28. A	41. B	54. D
3. D	16. C	29. A	42. C	55. A
4. C	17. B	30. B	43. C	56. B
5. A	18. D	31. A	44. A	57. C
6. B	19. D	32. C	45. D	58. A
7. B	20. A	33. C	46. A	59. B
8. D	21. D	34. C	47. C	60. D
9. A	22. C	35. A	48. B	61. C
10. A	23. C	36. D	49. D	62. D
11. D	24. D	37. A	50. A	63. C
12. B	25. C	38. B	51. B	64. B
13. B	26. C	39. D	52. A	65. D

ANATOMY AND PHYSIOLOGY

1. A	16. D	31. B	46. D	61. B
2. D	17. C	32. B	47. A	62. C
3. A	18. B	33. C	48. A	63. C
4. C	19. D	34. C	49. A	64. B
5. A	20. C	35. D	50. B	65. B
6. B	21. B	36. C	51. C	66. B
7. A	22. B	37. B	52. B	67. C
8. B	23. A	38. A	53. B	68. B
9. A	24. C	39. A	54. D	69. D
10. D	25. B	40. D	55. D	70. B
11. A	26. D	41. B	56. B	71. A
12. C	27. C	42. A	57. C	72. A
13. A	28. C	43. D	58. B	73. C
14. A	29. A	44. B	59. B	74. D
15. D	30. D	45. D	60. B	75. C

BASICS OF CHEMISTRY AND ELECTRICITY

1. A	11. A	21. B	31. A	41. C
2. A	12. D	22. A	32. A	42. C
3. A	13. B	23. D	33. A	43. C
4. C	14. A	24. C	34. C	44. C
5. A	15. D	25. B	35. A	45. A
6. A	16. C	26. A	36. B	46. B
7. A	17. B	27. C	37. B	47. A
8. C	18. C	28. D	38. C	48. A
9. A	19. C	29. A	39. C	49. C
10. B	20. C	30. B	40. D	50. B

PROPERTIES OF THE HAIR AND SCALP

1. C	19. A	37. A	55. A	73. B
2. A	20. A	38. C	56. B	74. D
3. D	21. C	39. B	57. C	75. A
4. C	22. D	40. C	58. C	76. D
5. D	23. D	41. C	59. A	77. D
6. B	24. C	42. C	60. D	78. C
7. D	25. C	43. B	61. B	79. D
8. C	26. B	44. D	62. B	80. B
9. D	27. D	45. A	63. A	81. B
10. C	28. C	46. B	64. B	82. A
11. D	29. A	47. D	65 D	83. B
12. D	30. A	48. A	66. D	84. B
13. C	31. D	49. C	67. A	85. B
14. B	32. C	50. A	68. B	86. B
15. D	33. D	51. B	69. C	87. C
16. B	34. A	52. C	70. C	88. C
17. C	35. B	53. D	71. C	89. D
18. D	36. A	54. B	72. C	90. A

PRINCIPLES OF HAIR DESIGN

1. C	9. B	17. B	25. D	33. B
2. A	10. A	18. D	26. C	34. A
3. B	11. D	19. D	27. D	35. A
4. B	12. C	20. C	28. D	36. B
5. B	13. D	21. A	29. A	37. D
6. D	14. A	22. B	30. D	38. D
7. B	15. B	23. A	31. A	39. D
8. A	16. C	24. A	32. D	40. A

SHAMPOOING, RINSING, AND CONDITIONING

1. D	13. D	25. A	37. B	49. A
2. D	14. D	26. A	38. D	50. C
3. D	15. B	27. C	39. B	51. C
4. C	16. D	28. B	40. B	52. C
5. A	17. B	29. C	41. C	53. A
6. D	18. B	30. A	42. A	54. D
7. B	19. D	31. D	43. B	55. D
8. A	20. B	32. B	44. A	56. B
9. A	21. A	33. D	45. D	57. A
10. A	22. B	34. D	46. A	58. A
11. D	23. A	35. A	47. C	59. C
12. D	24. A	36. B	48. C	60. D

HAIRCUTTING

1. A	16. D	31. A	46. C	61. B
2. A	17. A	32. A	47. A	62. C
3. C	18. D	33. D	48. C	63. B
4. B	19. C	34. D	49. C	64. B
5. B	20. D	35. A	50. C	65. C
6. B	21. D	36. C	51. A	66. B
7. D	22. A	37. C	52. B	67. C
8. A	23. A	38. B	53. A	68. A
9. C	24. A	39. D	54. D	69. C
10. D	25. B	40. D	55. D	70. C
11. D	26. A	41. A	56. D	71. C
12. D	27. B	42. A	57. A	72. D
13. C	28. B	43. C	58. A	73. C
14. A	29. D	44. D	59. A	74. A
15. D	30. C	45. D	60. B	75. B

HAIRSTYLING

1. A	21. B	41. B	61. D	81. C
2. C	22. C	42. C	62. B	82. D
3. D	23. A	43. A	63. A	83. A
4. B	24. B	44. C	64. B	84. B
5. A	25. C	45. A	65. D	85. C
6. D	26. D	46. C	66. B	86. D
7. A	27. B	47. D	67. C	87. A
8. C	28. D	48. C	68. D	88. B
9. D	29. C	49. A	69. C	89. A
10. C	30. D	50. B	70. B	90. C
11. A	31. B	51. D	71. C	91. B
12. B	32. A	52. B	72. A	92. A
13. C	33. D	53. C	73. B	93. C
14. D	34. B	54. D	74. A	94. B
15. C	35. D	55. B	75. D	95. C
16. D	36. C	56. D	76. A	96. D
17. B	37. A	57. A	77. C	97. B
18. A	38. D	58. D	78. A	98. A
19. D	39. C	59. A	79. D	99. D
20. C	40. A	60. B	80. B	100. B

BRAIDING AND BRAID EXTENSIONS

1. A	5. B	9. A	13. D	17. C
2. C	6. D	10. C	14. B	18. B
3. D	7. B	11. D	15. D	19. D
4. A	8. C	12. A	16. A	20. C

WIGS AND HAIR ENHANCEMENTS

1. A	7. D	13. B	19. C	25. C
2. D	8. A	14. A	20. D	26. A
3. B	9. C	15. C	21. C	27. B
4. D	10. B	16. B	22. A	28. D
5. B	11. A	17. D	23. D	29. A
6. A	12. C	18. B	24. A	30. C

CHEMICAL TEXTURE SERVICES

1. B	20. A	39. C	58. B	77. C
2. C	21. D	40. A	59. D	78. A
3. D	22. A	41. D	60. A	79. B
4. A	23. D	42. C	61. D	80. C
5. B	24. B	43. D	62. C	81. D
6. C	25. C	44. B	63. D	82. B
7. D	26. D	45. C	64. C	83. A
8. B	27. A	46. B	65. D	84. D
9. C	28. D	47. A	66. B	85. C
10. D	29. B	48. D	67. A	86. A
11. B	30. C	49. A	68. D	87. C
12. C	31. D	50. D	69. C	88. A
13. A	32. A	51. A	70. B	89. B
14. B	33. C	52. C	71. D	90. A
15. A	34. D	53. D	72. C	91. B
16. D	35. A	54. B	73. B	92. D
17. B	36. B	55. C	74. D	93. A
18. D	37. A	56. A	75. A	94. D
19. C	38. D	57. A	76. D	95. B

HAIRCOLORING

1. D	20. D	39. B	58. A	77. B
2. B	21. C	40. D	59. C	78. D
3. D	22. A	41. B	60. D	79. B
4. A	23. D	42. C	61. B	80. A
5. C	24. C	43. A	62. D	81. C
6. B	25. D	44. D	63. A	82. D
7. A	26. A	45. C	64. D	83. B
8. D	27. D	46. B	65. C	84. A
9. B	28. A	47. C	66. B	85. D
10. A	29. B	48. B	67. A	86. B
11. D	30. C	49. C	68. D	87. A
12. C	31. B	50. D	69. B	88. C
13. A	32. A	51. C	70. A	89. A
14. C	33. D	52. D	71. B	90. B
15. B	34. B	53. C	72. D	91. A
16. A	35. D	54. A	73. C	
17. D	36. C	55. B	74. B	
18. C	37. D	56. C	75. C	
19. B	38. C	57. D	76. A	

HISTOLOGY OF THE SKIN

1. B	17. B	33. B	49. B	65. B
2. C	18. D	34. C	50. A	66. A
3. A	19. C	35. D	51. C	67. B
4. B	20. A	36. A	52. A	68. D
5. D	21. C	37. B	53. B	69. A
6. B	22. D	38. D	54. C	70. B
7. A	23. A	39. C	55. B	71. C
8. D	24. C	40. D	56. A	72. B
9. B	25. D	41. B	57. C	73. A
10. D	26. C	42. C	58. C	74. C
11. B	27. B	43. A	59. A	75. A
12. C	28. C	44. D	60. D	76. C
13. B	29. A	45. A	61. B	77. D
14. C	30. B	46. C	62. D	78. A
15. D	31. A	47. B	63. A	79. C
16. A	32. C	48. C	64. D	80. A

HAIR REMOVAL

1. C	6. D	11. B	16. D	21. C
2. B	7. A	12. D	17. C	22. A
3. D	8. D	13. C	18. A	23. B
4. B	9. A	14. D	19. B	24. A
5. A	10. C	15. B	20. A	

FACIALS

1. D	15. B	29. C	43. B	57. C
2. A	16. C	30. B	44. C	58. B
3. C	17. D	31. D	45. D	59. D
4. D	18. C	32. B	46. A	60. C
5. B	19. D	33. A	47. C	61. B
6. D	20. B	34. D	48. A	62. A
7. B	21. C	35. B	49. C	63. B
8. D	22. D	36. A	50. B	64. A
9. B	23. C	37. C	51. C	65. B
10. D	24. A	38. A	52. A	66. C
11. C	25. C	39. B	53. D	67. D
12. B	26. D	40. C	54. B	68. C
13. C	27. C	41. A	55. A	69. A
14. A	28. A	42. C	56. B	70. D

FACIAL MAKEUP

1. A	7. D	13. B	19. A	25. D
2. C	8. C	14. A	20. C	26. A
3. B	9. A	15. C	21. B	27. C
4. A	10. C	16. A	22. D	28. A
5. D	11. B	17. B	23. B	29. D
6. A	12. C	18. C	24. A	30. B

NAIL STRUCTURE AND GROWTH

1. C	11. C	21. A	31. D	41. D
2. A	12. D	22. B	32. A	42. C
3. B	13. C	23. C	33. C	43. A
4. A	14. D	24. B	34. B	44. B
5. D	15. B	25. C	35. A	45. C
6. C	16. A	26. D	36. C	46. D
7. B	17. B	27. B	37. A	47. B
8. C	18. D	28. D	38. D	48. A
9. B	19. B	29. B	39. A	49. D
10. A	20. B	30. A	40. C	50. C

MANICURING AND PEDICURING

1. B	9. D	17. D	25. C	33. C
2. C	10. C	18. B	26. D	34. D
3. B	11. D	19. A	27. B	35. B
4. A	12. A	20. C	28. C	36. D
5. D	13. D	21. D	29. D	37. C
6. A	14. C	22. C	30. A	38. D
7. C	15. D	23. D	31. D	39. A
8. D	16. C	24. B	32. A	40. D

ADVANCED NAIL TECHNIQUES

1. B	6. A	11. B	16. D	21. D
2. C	7. D	12. C	17. A	22. C
3. B	8. C	13. A	18. D	23. D
4. C	9. D	14. C	19. B	24. C
5. D	10. C	15. B	20. C	25. B

THE SALON BUSINESS

1. D	9. C	17. A	25. D	33. C
2. B	10. B	18. B	26. A	34. D
3. A	11. A	19. D	27. B	35. B
4. D	12. B	20. C	28. A	36. C
5. B	13. A	21. B	29. D	37. A
6. A	14. B	22. A	30. C	38. D
7. C	15. A	23. C	31. D	39. A
8. B	16. D	24. B	32. B	40. D

SEEKING EMPLOYMENT

1. C	6. C	11. D	16. B	21. C
2. B	7. B	12. A	17. D	22. D
3. A	8. C	13. C	18. A	23. A
4. C	9. D	14. B	19. D	24. B
5. A	10. B	15. A	20. B	25. A

ON THE JOB

1. D	6. A	11. D	16. C	21. B
2. A	7. D	12. C	17. D	22. D
3. C	8. B	13. A	18. C	23. A
4. D	9. C	14. C	19. D	24. B
5. B	10. A	15. D	20. C	25. C